Health Informatics

Kathryn J. Hannah   Marion J. Ball
Series Editors

Springer
New York
Berlin
Heidelberg
Barcelona
Hong Kong
London
Milan
Paris
Singapore
Tokyo

Health Informatics Series
(formerly Computers in Health Care)

Series Editors
Kathryn J. Hannah   Marion J. Ball

(continued after Index)

Naakesh A. Dewan   Nancy M. Lorenzi
Robert T. Riley   Sarbori R. Bhattacharya
Editors

Behavorial Healthcare
Informatics

With a Foreword by Howard H. Goldman, M.D., Ph.D.

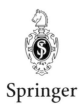

Springer

Naakesh A. Dewan, M.D.
Executive Director
Center for Quality
  Innovations & Research
Department of Psychiatry
University of Cincinnati
Cincinnati, OH 45219-8048,
USA

Nancy M. Lorenzi Ph.D.
Professor and Assistant
  Vice Chancellor
  for Health Affairs
Vanderbilt University
  Medical Center
Nashville, TN 37232-8340,
USA

Robert T. Riley, Ph.D.
President
Riley Associates
Nashville, TN 37215,
USA

Sarbori R. Bhattacharya, M.D.
Resident Physician
Department of Psychiatry
University of Cincinnati
Cincinnati, OH 45219-8048
USA

Series Editors:
Kathryn J. Hannah,
  Ph.D., R.N.
Professor, Department of
  Community Health
  Science
Faculty of Medicine
The University of Calgary
Calgary, Alberta, Canada

Marion J. Ball, Ed.D.
Adjunct Professor
Johns Hopkins University
  School of Nursing
formerly
Vice President
First Consulting Group
Baltimore, MD 21210
USA

Cover illustration ©2001 Artville, Inc.
With 7 illustrations

R A 790. 5
, B 36 5
2 0 0 2

Library of Congress Cataloging-in-Publication Data
Behavioral healthcare informatics / edited by Naakesh A. Dewan . . . [et al.]
    p. ; cm.—(Health informatics)
    ISBN 0-387-95265-9 (h/c : alk. paper)
    1. Managed mental health care. 2. Medical informatics. I. Dewan, Naakesh A. II.
Series
    [DNLM: 1. Behavorial Medicine—organization & administration. 2. Managed Care
    Programs—organization & administration. 3. Medical Informatics. WB 103 B4195 2001]
    RA790.5 .B365 2001
    362.2–dc21   2001020192

Printed on acid-free paper.

Production managed by Terry Kornak; manufacturing supervised by Erica Bresler.
Typeset by Matrix Publishing Services, York, PA.
Printed and bound by Edwards Brothers, Inc., Ann Arbor, MI.
Printed in the United States of America.

9 8 7 6 5 4 3 2 1

ISBN 0-387-95265-9   SPIN 107997803

Springer-Verlag   New York Berlin Heidelberg
A member of BertelsmannSpringer Science+Business Media GmbH

This book is dedicated to the people whose support, love, and encouragement have been essential to the success of my efforts. To Nancy Lorenzi, my informatics guru, for her mentorship and unselfishness. To my father, Amrit L. Dewan, a world-class athlete and information systems analyst, who taught me to always strive for the very best in all endeavors. To my mother, Gopi Dewan, a physician, who showed me the joy of healing and caring for others. To my sons, Ashwin and Shyam, for reminding me every day what is really important in life. Finally, to my wife, Devaki, a radiologist with boundless energy, whose love, sacrifice, and daily support and encouragement make life wonderful and all dreams possible.

Naakesh A. Dewan

We dedicate this book to all the behavioral and informatics pioneers who are helping to create a better future.

Nancy M. Lorenzi and Robert T. Riley

"It takes a village to raise a child." I would like to dedicate my first work to the village chiefs, Drs. Naakesh Dewan and Nancy Lorenzi, for giving me the opportunity to write a dedication in the first place. Then, of course, there are my parents, Amar and Minati Bhattacharya, whose guidance, love, and unending quest for knowledge kept me from being the village idiot. Next is the village doctor, who also happens to be my husband, Sambhu Choudhury. His support, wisdom, and generosity mean the world to me, and I would not be where or who I am today without him. Finally, there are my friends, who made my village the best one on the planet. Lali, Deepak, Arturo, Diana, and Karen, thanks for all your patience and encouragement.

Sarbori R. Bhattacharya

Foreword

Mental Health: A Report of the Surgeon General underscores the need for a volume on behavioral informatics without mentioning the field by name even once.

The bulk of the 500 pages of the first-ever report from the surgeon general is devoted to the advances in science in the mental health field. It places mental health within the mainstream of health, as a fundamental component of individual well-being. The report details the evidence for the effectiveness of mental health treatments and services. Further, the report encourages Americans to seek help and to fight the stigma associated with mental illness. The surgeon general identifies the gap between the potential of science and the reality of limited access and actual practice as a serious problem for mental health policy to address. All of these issues turn on the availability of information and a set of techniques and specifications for storing, sharing, and using it. At one level that involves data from research. At another level it means information for service delivery and decision making. The benefits of science and effective treatment cannot be accomplished without a strong information base. Consequently, we need a science of informatics to guide our choices and our decisions. A definitive book like *Behavioral Healthcare Informatics* is an important contribution, because it supports research and practice.

The report of the surgeon general also cautioned about the threats to privacy and confidentiality in the information age. A chapter was devoted to this topic, expressing concern that a loss of confidentiality might threaten the trust needed for individuals with a mental health problem or mental disorder to overcome the stigma and their resistance and to seek treatment.

As a society we must resolve the tension between the promise of information and the threat to privacy posed by its ready availability. We need a technology to make information more accessible and more quickly available to provide better care and treatment to individuals troubled by mental disorders and mental health problems. But individuals must feel comfortable coming forward to receive that care. Confidentiality is essential to the process. Resolving these tensions is a critical step toward better mental health.

This new book, *Behavioral Healthcare Informatics*, written by experts with a concern for technology and humanity, is a dramatic step in the right direction. It will be useful to service users and service providers, researchers and clinicians, as well as program managers and policy makers.

Howard H. Goldman, M.D., Ph.D.
Scientific Editor, *Mental Health: A Report of the Surgeon General*
Professor of Psychiatry
University of Maryland School of Medicine
Baltimore, Maryland

Series Preface

This series is directed to healthcare professionals who are leading the transformation of health care by using information and knowledge. Launched in 1988 as Computers in Health Care, the series offers a broad range of titles: some addressed to specific professions such as nursing, medicine, and health administration; others to special areas of practice such as trauma and radiology. Still other books in the series focus on interdisciplinary issues, such as the computer-based patient record, electronic health records, and networked healthcare systems.

Renamed Health Informatics in 1998 to reflect the rapid evolution in the discipline now known as health informatics, the series will continue to add titles that contribute to the evolution of the field. In the series, eminent experts, serving as editors or authors, offer their accounts of innovations in health informatics. Increasingly, these accounts go beyond hardware and software to address the role of information in influencing the transformation of healthcare delivery systems around the world. The series also increasingly focuses on "peopleware" and the organizational, behavioral, and societal changes that accompany the diffusion of information technology in health services environments.

These changes will shape health services in this new millennium. By making full and creative use of the technology to tame data and to transform information, health informatics will foster the development of the knowledge age in health care. As coeditors, we pledge to support our professional colleagues and the series readers as they share advances in the emerging and exciting field of health informatics.

Kathryn J. Hannah
Marion J. Ball

Preface

In a recent report sponsored by the World Health Organization and the World Bank, behavioral health disorders combined accounted for almost half of the top ten causes of disease burden worldwide. Informatics is just beginning to transform behavioral health and care as it has transformed medical and surgical care. Nowhere else can a little investment in information technology research and development mean so much for so many worldwide. The promise and future of behavioral informatics is outlined in the chapters that follow.

The book is divided into sections that can serve as "modules" for the reader. Sections cover both the science and practice of clinical computing, consumer informatics, quality, technological issues, and organizational imperatives. The authors are physicians, psychologists, informatics executives, researchers, engineers, and sociologists. This diversity of perspectives brings richness to the book and will keep the reader interested and focused.

In the first section, the editors overview the entire landscape of behavioral informatics, which is then followed by a simple, yet comprehensive, chapter on the technologies that will support the convergence of behavioral health care and informatics. The next section covers the entire array of emerging clinical technologies from psychotherapy, to medication management, to care management. The third section focuses on the impact of technology on quality in both the public and private sectors. The final section focuses on the organization and leaderships issues involved in transforming a behavioral healthcare organization into an e-behavioral healthcare organization.

In this book, Naakesh A. Dewan, M.D., a leader in behavioral informatics, managed care, and quality improvement, joins with Nancy Lorenzi, Ph.D., Robert Riley, Ph.D., and Sarbori Bhattacharya, M.D., in editing an essential book on behavioral informatics. The editors have crafted a book in collaboration with nationally recognized experts in the field to fill the discipline's tremendous void.

This book is essential for students and faculty in departments of psychiatry, psychology, social work, other human service disciplines, and informatics departments. It is for clinicians, administrators, information technology (IT) executives, and consumers who wish to know what is possible today and what lies ahead as both technology and behavioral health care converge.

We hope this book will be considered a "must read" in the field of health informatics. We feel that it is a necessary reference book for any educational, public, or personal library.

Naakesh A. Dewan
Nancy M. Lorenzi
Robert T. Riley
Sarbori R. Bhattacharya

Contents

PART III CONSUMERS' ISSUES

PART IV INFORMATICS AND QUALITY IMPROVEMENT

PART V ORGANIZATIONAL ISSUES

Contributors

Norman Alessi, M.D.
Associate Professor and Chief Information Officer, University of Michigan Department of Psychiatry, Ann Arbor, MI 48109, USA

Kenneth Z. Altshuler, M.D.
Professor Emeritus, Department of Psychiatry, University of Texas Southwestern Medical Center, Dallas, TX 75235, USA

Shannon M. Baker, M.A.
Research Assistant, University of Texas Southwestern Medical Center, Dallas, TX 75390-9101, USA

Suresh Bangara, M.D.
Founder and President, Integrated Health Partners, Woodinville, Washington; Assistant Professor, Clinical Department of Psychiatry and Behavioral Sciences, Koeck School of Medicine, University of Southern California, Los Angeles, CA 90033, USA

Sarbori R. Bhattacharya, M.D.
Resident Physician, Department of Psychiatry, University of Cincinnati College of Medicine, Cincinnati, OH 45219-8048, USA

Sara J. Czaja, Ph.D.
Professor of Engineering and Psychiatry, University of Miami; Director, Center for Research and Education on Aging and Technology Advancement (CREATE), Miami, FL 33136, USA

Les DelPizzo
Director, Strategic Sales, CMHC Systems, Inc., Dublin, OH 43017, USA

Naakesh A. Dewan, M.D.
Executive Director, Center for Quality Innovations & Research; Adjunct Assistant Clinical Professor of Psychiatry, University of Cincinnati College of Medicine, Cincinnati, OH 45219-8048, USA

William S. Edell, Ph.D.
Senior Vice President, Clinical Development Mental Health Outcomes, Inc., Horizon Health Corporation, Lewisville, TX 75057-6011

Howard Goldman, M.D., Ph.D.
Scientific Editor, *Mental Health: A Report of the Surgeon General*; Professor of Psychiatry, University of Maryland School of Medicine, Baltimore, MD 21201, USA

Ellen Graves
Marketing Manager, McKesson Clinical Reference Products, Broomfield, CO 80021, USA

Marilyn J. Henderson, Ph.D.
Assistant Chief, Survey and Analysis Branch, Center for Mental Health Services Administration, Rockville, MD 20857, USA

Milton Huang, M.D.
Assistant Director, University of Michigan Psychiatric Informatics Program; Lecturer, University of Michigan Department of Psychiatry, Ann Arbor, MI 48109, USA

Robert Kennedy, M.S.
Editor and Program Director of Medicine, Psychiatry, and Mental Health Division, Medscape, New York, NY 10001-4905, USA

Janet K. Kern, Ph.D., R.N.
Fellow, University of Texas Southwestern Medical Center, Dallas, TX 75390-9101, USA

Chin Chin Lee, M.S.
Research Fellow, Center for Research and Education on Aging and Technology Advancement (CREATE), University of Miami, Miami, FL 33136, USA

Nancy M. Lorenzi, Ph.D.
Assistant Vice Chancellor for Health Affairs and, Professor of Biomedical Informatics, Vanderbilt University Medical Center, Nashville, TN 37232, USA

Ronald Manderscheid, M.D.
Chief, Survey and Analysis Branch, Center for Mental Health Services Administration, Rockville, MD 20857, USA

Ross D. Martin, M.D., MHA
Senior Manager, Business Technology, Pfizer Pharmaceuticals Group, New York, NY 10017, USA

Sarah L. Minden, M.D.
Assistant Professor of Psychiatry, Harvard Medical School, Boston, MA; Senior Scientist, Abt Associates, Cambridge, MA 02138-1168, USA

David Olson M.D., Ph.D.
Assistant Professor in Psychiatry, University of Massachusetts School of Medicine, Worcester, MA 01655, USA

Raymond L. Ownby, M.D., Ph.D.
Director, Geriatric Psychiatry Research, and Director, Cognitive Neuroscience Group, Department of Psychiatry and Behavioral Sciences, University of Miami, Miami, FL 33140-2800, USA

Robert T. Riley, Ph.D.
President, Riley Associates, Nashville, TN 37215, USA

Charles Ruetsch, Ph.D.
Senior Scientist, IMR, an AdvancePCS Company, Hunt Valley, MD 21031, USA

Richard Thompson
Vice President, McKesson Clinical Reference Products, Broomfield, CO 80021, USA

Madhukar H. Trivedi, M.D.
Director, Depression and Anxiety Disorders Program; Associate Professor, University of Texas Southwestern Medical Center, Dallas, TX 75390-9101, USA

Tracy M. Voegtle, M.A.
Research Assistant, University of Texas Southwestern Medical Center, Dallas, TX 75390-9101, USA

David M. Wadell, M.S.
Vice President Quality Improvement, Workplace Group, Magellan Behavioral Health, Columbia, MD 21046, USA

Lawrence G. Weiss, Ph.D., M.S.
Director of Behavioral Healthcare and Personality Group, Psychological Corporation, San Antonio, TX 78204-2498, USA

Part I
Overview

1
Behavioral Health and Informatics: An Overview

Naakesh A. Dewan, Nancy M. Lorenzi, Robert T. Riley, and Sarbori R. Bhattacharya

The $99 billion behavioral health industry has gone through dramatic changes during the last decade. Managed behavioral care systems have grown from covering 60 million people to covering over 170 million in the United States. At the same time, 23 states have received waivers from the federal government to transform Medicaid fee-for-service care into managed care delivery systems. This trend will spread to all 50 states and five territories of the United States. Over 2,000 federally funded community mental health centers are also embracing transforming information technologies.

There are over 5,000 organizations providing behavioral health services in the United States. These organizations include group practices, hospital-based delivery systems, community mental health centers, and medical hospitals providing behavioral health services through partnerships with behavioral health entities. One common theme in the alteration of the financing and delivery of behavioral health care has been the need for information technologies and systems that can transform the access to, coordination of, and accountability of these systems of care.

The behavioral healthcare industry has suffered the same perception of payers as the medical and surgical industry: a tremendous amount of money is spent with limited value and accountability. Throughout this book, examples and trends in the field of informatics are reviewed and discussed. These examples provide the reader with a demonstration of the enabling power of information systems to drive the transformation of the delivery of health care, and to help healthcare systems achieve the goals of access, affordability, and accountability.

In the clinical arena, the advances in information technology have included computerized assessment tools and the development of manual-based psychotherapies, which have been transformed into computerized-based psychotherapies. There are now computerized therapies for depression, anxiety, and stress management, and emerging computerized initiatives in manual-based addiction treatment and schizophrenia will surely come of age in the next 5 years. Medication algorithms have also been computerized.

The field of behavioral health care has always emphasized, in both psychology and psychiatry, the need to codify and quantify the diagnosis, the severity of illness, and the need for treatment. A plethora of psychometric instruments exists to help clinicians evaluate and treat consumers in distress who are seeking behavioral health services. These instruments are now available either in software packages or over the Internet.

Clinical decision support systems, however, had not been the focus of behavioral health care until recently. Thus, the behavioral healthcare field is significantly behind the surgical and medical informatics field in this area and in accessing knowledge at the point of care. However, computer-assisted assessment systems are now available. Given the rich system of psychometric measurement in the behavioral healthcare field, these systems will soon be the norm in practice settings.

Organizations as well as clinicians are being impacted by information technology. Beginning in 1990, the behavioral healthcare field embraced the concept of outcomes measurement. Today, over 75 companies in the United States sell clinical assessment and outcome measurement tools. The specific event that created such a growth in this outcomes measurement industry was the mandate by the Joint Commission on Accreditation of Healthcare Organizations to require accredited healthcare organizations to have a performance measurement system in place. Over the next few years there will certainly be consolidation in this field as mergers and acquisitions occur. Depending on industry trends and requirements, changing regulations may demand less or more in performance measurement.

During the past decade, there has been growth in the managed care systems that offer and sell greater access, affordability, and accountability to payers, and clinician and professional profiling has become the norm. This profiling pertains mostly to administrative data rather than to clinical data, for example, the average number of visits to an outpatient setting, or the average number of days spent in an inpatient setting. Multiple challenges exist in the private sector to integrate diverse data sets and applications.

In the public sector there has been a 20-year trend to develop, through the mental health statistics improvement program, information systems that support performance measurement and accountability. Unfortunately, federal standards are often refined and customized at both the state and community levels, yielding disparate ways of collecting, analyzing, and representing data at over 2,000 community mental health centers in the United States. The emphasis on getting local stakeholder buy-in versus creating a national standard is a debate not only in health care but also in all sectors of the U.S. economy (e.g., education, tax codes, or laws about speed limits). New federal initiatives are once again being promulgated with the hopes of establishing a uniform decision support vehicle.

Another recent trend in the clinical area has been the development of clinical prescription systems. Both physicians and consumer advocates have raised a number of concerns. The pharmaceutical industry and pharmacists around the country are pushing for on-line prescriptions. The backdrop for this is a struggle for professional "turfs," where maintaining the physician–patient relationship and human contact is seen as an essential part of treatment. The Internet and other information technologies—telephonic prescriptions, mail-order prescriptions—replace that human interface. The capacity of on-line prescriptions and remote pre-scription systems pressures professionals into thinking "out of the box." Utilizing technologies to complement current practice is the major dilemma for the field.

The introduction of information technology in the clinical area has raised a number of ethical concerns. Behavioral health care has prided itself on treating every patient as an individual with unique needs, perspectives, and backgrounds. But quantified assessment treatment-monitoring systems tend to reduce the per-ceived influence of the clinician. Mandatory sharing of information with payers has continued to be a problematic area.

The past decade has seen dramatic changes in hardware, applications, and com-munications technology. The Internet, since 1990, has grown at an exponential rate, as has the number of Web sites. The use of Internet technology has out-paced the use of previous technologies, such as the telephone, VCRs, and DVD systems. As chip capacity grows every 6 months, application and software de-velopment capacity also grows. This creates a tremendous burden on both the purchaser and user of behavioral health information systems. The growth in com-munication tools and the growing capacity of existing hardware to handle a tremendous amount of data traffic, including full-screen video, will be changing the way remote-site learning and "distance therapy" are conducted. Technolo-gies for interactive voice recognition systems will be able to detect subtle changes in voice patterns and to determine the affect state of the speaker, and thus add both knowledge and confusion to the behavioral health landscape. Optical fiber and switch technology will make "terabyte" (1 trillion bytes) traffic possible.

There are, of course, tremendous risks in technology innovation. The problem with rapid advancement is that there is not enough time to study and evaluate a given technology to ascertain whether it is reliable and valid, and whether it is used in similar ways across patients and across treatment settings. This variation in the use and adaptation of technology will continue to add variation to the de-livery of health care, which is a fundamental quality issue that all healthcare sys-tems face. While it is somewhat cumbersome and rudimentary to develop stan-dards, they are greatly needed in behavioral healthcare information technology. The medical and surgical world has gone through these standards development processes, and behavioral health care needs to begin this journey.

Information technology and the rapid evolution of communications, hardware, and software capacity will greatly improve the ability to design and implement sys-tems of care. Managed care will continue to grow. Definitive partnerships and col-laborations between payers, insurers, and providers must be established. While there may be differences in terms of risk sharing, reimbursement rates, and provider and network makeup, it will be essential to have a common language and common data standards to ensure that the public receives efficient and cost-effective care.

Unfortunately, planning such large-scale implementations takes more time than is available in today's behavioral healthcare marketplace. There will certainly be some very difficult and painful experiences noticed by a number of organiza-tions. While the redesign of the financing and structure of behavioral health care moves rapidly, the use of information technology has been an opportunity either to buffer that tremendous change or to cause even more stress. It will be essential to have very detailed and crisp systems and information technology (IT) planning in these new behavioral healthcare environments. Enabling technologies such as XML (extensible markup language) will allow disparate systems to talk to each other. XML is the emerging standard for defining, transmitting, validating, and transmitting data over the Internet.

The acceptance of information technology in research areas has proven that failure is due not to the technology but rather to the inability of individuals in organizations to provide input and to work with each other. It is the behavioral health field that has impacted medical and surgical fields in the informatics area and that has fostered the organizational psychology of systems. Behavioral health care has always been an interdisciplinary environment, and it has the ability to foster greater acceptance of information technology.

Another area where advances in technology can greatly benefit and improve the quality of healthcare for individuals suffering from mental illness is in education and research. Standardized patient psychotherapies can greatly enhance the problem-solving skills and education of professionals. There will be a tremendous boom in the development of central nervous system (CNS) medications in the next 5 years. The amount and quantity of information available will be exponentially greater than what has been available in the psychiatrist's armamentarium in the past four decades.

This explosion in the new sciences and in medication development will put increased stresses on the knowledge demands of all professionals. The technologies, especially the Internet technologies, that make knowledge available are credible and easy to use, but must be frequently updated.

Traditional information systems have always been used for back-office functions. Information technology, historically on a national scale, has expanded from national security, to financial and banking systems, and finally to entertainment. Now in health care the same kinds of progression are evolving, where technology is used for ensuring the security and financial survivability of an organization. However, due to the growing demand of quality accountability, coordination, and access to care issues that are prevalent in the 21st century, systems must be able to provide real-time knowledge and decision support as well as ongoing strategic decision support for both clinicians and administrators.

There are several ways that information technology can improve quality of care. This book reviews a number of outcomes measurement technologies, communication technologies that enhance access to care, and smart cards in electronic medical records that allow ongoing communication across disparate settings.

Historically, the emphasis in the 1960s and 1970s was placed on structure, in the 1980s on process, and in the 1990s on outcomes. Outcomes research integrated with structural and process research will dominate in the 21st century. Qualitative research and research that goes on outside of the actual setting of data capture are also important, but they will not receive the amount of financial support they have previously. Behavioral health care, just like any field in health care, is a mixture of art and science. There are times when not all data are capturable through quantitative needs.

Impact Issues

The behavioral health technology movement will significantly impact the knowledge base and knowledge delivery vehicles for all those involved in behavioral health care, from consumer to provider to payer to insurer. Given the tremendous diversity of organizations providing behavioral health care, knowledge will be gained through how different sectors of the behavioral healthcare economy respond to technologies. Questions regarding the differences between community mental health centers, private group practices, managed behavior companies, and hospitals will be developed. This knowledge will be essential in terms of efficient and effective implementation of technologies in these settings.

One of the biggest dilemmas in the behavioral healthcare arena, especially due to the recent policy mandates of integration with medical care, is information privacy, specifically mental health privacy. While there may be a need for a primary care physician to understand the medical and some of the psychiatric aspects of the patient being treated in behavioral healthcare, practitioners are resistant to sharing this information. Unfortunately, this resistance contributes to patients' perceptions of behavioral healthcare practitioners as untrustworthy and lacking value. It will require a great deal of organizational group processes and organizational change strategies to implement these technological systems.

In summary, behavioral health care is unique in the medical field. The communication that goes on between provider and patient forms a great part of the therapy. This is unlike any other specialty in health care. The approach by a therapist to search, dissect, discover, and treat the pains of the past and present will surely be enhanced by the adoption of information technology in the new millennium.

Bibliography

Amatayakul M. Achieving compliance with the new standards. *MD Comput* 2000;17(3): 54–55.

Amatayakul M. Security and privacy in the health information age. *MD Comput* 1999; 16(6):51–53.

Anderson JG, Brann M. Security of medical information: the threat from within. *MD Comput* 2000;17:(2):15–17.

Brennan PF. Knowing what to do: international perspectives on the roles of clinical guidelines and patient preferences in patient care. *JAMIA* 1998;5(3);317–318.

Buckovich SA, Rippen HE, Rozen MJ. Driving toward guiding principles: a goal for privacy, confidentiality, and security of health information. *JAMIA* 1999;6(2):122–133.

Chute CG, Cohn SP, Campbell JR. A framework for comprehensive health terminology systems in the United States: development guidelines, criteria for selection, and public policy implications. *JAMIA* 1998;5(6):503–510.

Collen MF. The Internet and the World Wide Web. *MD Comput* 1999;16(5):72.

Collen MF. The origins of informatics. *MD Comput* 1999;16(1):104.

Collen MF. A vision of health care and informatics in 2008. *JAMIA* 1999;6(1):1–5.

Dick RS, Steen EB. eds. Committee on Improving the Patient Record. *The Computer-*

Based Patient Record: An Essential Technology for Health Care. National Academy Press, Washington, DC 1991. Division of Health Care Services, Institute of Medicine, 1991.

Dorenfest S. *The decade of the 90's.* Healthcare Informatics August 2000;64–67.

Greenes RA, Lorenzi NM. Audacious goals for health and biomedical informatics in the new millennium. *JAMIA* 1998;5(5):395–400.

Greist JH, Jefferson JW, Wenzel KW, et al. The telephone assessment program: efficient patient monitoring and clinician feedback. *MD Comput* 1997;14(5):382–387.

Johnshoy-Currie CJ. Stepping up to the challenge. *MD Comput* 2000;17(1):19.

Kane B, Sands DZ. Guidelines for the clinical use of electronic mail with patients. *JAMIA* 1998;5(1):104–111.

Lewis D. Computer-based approaches to patient education: a review of the literature. *JAMIA* 1999;6(4):272–282.

Mental Health, United States, 1998. DHHS publication no. (SMA) 99-3285. Washington, DC: Center for Mental Health Services, 1998.

Meyeroff WJ, Meyeroff RE. Behavior's problem. *Healthcare Informatics* 1999;16(3):59–65.

Rodsjo S. Prescribing information: no waiting on the Web. *Healthcare Informatics* 2000;17(4):133–138.

Rodsjo S. A progressive vision for progressive times. *Healthcare Informatics* August 2000;47–52.

Shaw SC, Marks IM, Toole S. Lessons from pilot tests of computer self-help for agora/claustrophobia and panic. *MD Comput* 2000;17(1):44–48.

Shiffman RN, Brandt CA, Liaw Y, Corb GJ. A design model for computer-based guideline implementation based on information management services. *JAMIA* 1999;6(2):99–103.

Shiffman RN, Liaw Y, Brandt CA, Corb GJ. Computer-based guideline implementation systems: a systematic review of functionality and effectiveness. *JAMIA* 1999;6(2):104–114.

Tang PC, Newcomb C. Informing patients: a guide for providing patient health information. *JAMIA* 1998;5(6):563–570.

Tange HJ, Schouten HC, Kester ADM, Hasman A. The granularity of medical narratives and its effect on the speed and completeness of information retrieval. *JAMIA* 1998;5(6):571–582.

U.S. Department of Health and Human Services. *Mental Health: A Report of the Surgeon General.* Rockville, MD: U.S. Department of Health and Human Services, Substance Abuse and Mental Health Services Administration, Center for Mental Health Services, National Institutes of Health, National Institute of Mental Health, 1999.

Van Bemmel JH. Privacy matters: who has the right to patient data? *MD Comput* 1999;16(5):21.

2
Technology Infrastructures

David Olson

Technological Systems

It is a strange fact that the healthcare industry as a whole, which represents approximately 7% of the United States economy, and the behavioral healthcare industry in particular have been extraordinarily slow to adopt the use of information systems for the coordination and delivery of their chief service—patient care. Financial and administrative functions including human resources, billing, and claims handling have long been processed, at least in part, by computer. Even these business functions, however, largely proceed via written records and paper-based transactions with insurance companies and data clearinghouses.

It is hard to find another sector of industry delivering services as complex and vital as medical or behavioral health care that utilizes information technology so ineffectively. It is often easier for a mental health care provider to go on-line to get instant data on the location and delivery status of an overnight package than it is to obtain data on past medication trials of an antidepressant from a patient's medical record. While many healthcare professionals view the business process as separate from, and indeed secondary to, the provision of quality care, this distinction is artificial. In addition to the traditional billing, claims processing, and accounts receivable functions, effective information system support of behavioral healthcare delivery requires integration of clinical data.

In an era of increasing delivery costs, declining reimbursement, and growing pressure to reduce expenses, the financial viability of a healthcare provider or behavioral system may depend critically on the ability to understand the factors that affect the cost of providing services. Decision support systems can integrate financial, clinical, and demographic data to help track, in real time, the changes in costs of providing care to a changing population. Analysis of these data can indicate changes in the severity and types of mental illness treated, the payer mix and rates of reimbursement by diagnostic category, and the referral sources.

Historically, information systems in behavioral health care have supported only core business functions such as billing and claims processing. The only clinical data stored in these systems are the procedure and diagnostic codes necessary to charge for services provided. These "legacy systems" remain in place throughout the country. In many offices, clinics, and hospitals, they remain the only electronically stored clinical data.

The utilization of information technology in behavioral health care is now beginning to change rapidly. Clinical information systems that support the delivery of behavioral health care and that contain large, longitudinal databases, which approximate or even replace the written medical record, are now becoming commercially available. Simultaneously, the technological infrastructure is evolving. Legacy systems such as the large mainframe and midrange computers, which have been the workhorses of the past two decades, are now being linked with, or replaced by, a host of specialized networked midrange and personal computer technology–based systems. The rapid development of network and distributed computing technology and operating systems software now provides the means for all computers, not just servers, on the network to both provide access to data and to share resources (scanners, backup devices, etc.) with other users. The means of accessing data from information systems by users has evolved from "dumb terminals" (with no processing capability) to personal computers and also wireless mobile hand-held computing devices. The explosive growth of the Internet and the availability of leased private high bandwidth (i.e., high data transmission rate) network connections (such as T1 and T3 lines) now allows for the components of distributed computing systems and databases to span the globe.

In behavioral health care, as in much of health care in general, we are currently in a transitional period. The information technology in use in the over 6,000 organizations providing behavioral health services in the United States varies widely. Paper-only systems abound, as do "big iron" central mainframe and midrange computer-based systems linked to end-users by dumb terminals (or personal computers emulating dumb terminals) and provide mainly billing, registration, and scheduling support. Information systems that utilize personal computers as clients and that access data from one or more "servers" (larger personal computers or midrange computer systems) are now relatively common and frequently coexist with legacy systems. These client/server-based systems have the advantage of sharing between the server and the client the work of managing the display and processing the data. Integrated systems linking legacy data with clinical or other data stored on networked servers are much less common. The newest and most flexible methodology for accessing data has its roots in the proliferation of the Internet and World Wide Web. Unlike client/server technology that requires application-specific software to be installed on every user's computer, the Web-based server approach requires only that an Internet browser such as Mosaic, Netscape, or Internet Explorer be installed. The server is responsible for all aspects of the data transaction from user authentication to the screen layout of the data to be displayed. A major advantage of the Web-based approach is that software upgrades need only to be deployed on the server and that any computer capable of running a browser, regardless of vendor, chip technology, or operating system, can access the server. Client-server based systems have the overhead of client software distribution and installation whenever the software is upgraded. One disadvantage of the Web-based approach is that the burden of most computational processing is shifted to the server.

Networks

A network is created by providing a means of communications between two or more computers. All computers on a network must be equipped with a network interface device that connects the computer to the network. The network connection may be over a coaxial cable, as in the case of Ethernet, a conventional or high-speed modem connection over a telephone line, or wireless communication medium such as infrared light, local or wide area radio broadcasting, or cellular telephone. Specialized high-speed network linkages are also widely available commercially from both telephone and cable service providers as well as specialized telecommunications companies.

In addition to the network interface electronics, software must be present on the computer that enables the operating system to interact with the network for the exchange of data. This software enables the computer to transmit and receive data using the appropriate network communication protocol. Various network protocols are in use around the world including Transmission Control Protocol/Internet Protocol (TCP/IP), Novell IPX (International Packet Exchange), AppleTalk, DECnet, and others. By far, the most common network protocol is TCP/IP, which is the standard for the Internet and World Wide Web. Data to be transmitted over the network is broken into small, sequential pieces called packets. In addition to the data, each packet has a "header," which contains the network addresses of both the originating and destination computer systems. In a large network, or in the case of the Internet, the packet may travel via many intermediate computer systems that serve as gateways (computers with multiple connections to other remote computer systems), which help to direct the data packet to its destination by the most efficient or available route. As the packets are received by the destination computer system, the data is reconstructed into its original form and processed or displayed by an application program such as a browser or specialized application program.

Networks provide connectivity between computer systems, creating the potential for messaging, data exchange, sharing of physical resources such as disk storage, backup devices, modems, and printers. Networked computers can work together combining computational power to perform large complex calculations, provided the task can be divided into pieces that can be worked on simultaneously. In this way, groups of small computers have been used to approximate the computational power of a large supercomputer. The Signs of Extraterrestrial Intelligence (SETI) @ Home project, for example, has used idle computer time on over 1.6 million computers in 224 countries to perform computer analysis of radio telescope data in the search for these signs. The amount of computing time contributed as of May 1999 was the equivalent of 165,000 years of supercomputer time averaging 10 trillion calculations per second (10 teraflops), 10 times more powerful than the largest supercomputer on the planet, and is the largest computation ever done.

As an example of a common network transaction, a mental health counselor might use the network connection of his personal computer in his office to access patient data from a centralized database system (on another floor of the building, or across town) by running an installed clinical information system program installed on his personal computer (PC). This program requests authentication in the form of a user name, password, and/or other validating information such as a thumbprint (biometric authentication), and presents this via the network for validation to the information system. Once authenticated, the counselor is granted access to the clinical database and may search for, retrieve, and display the requested information. When the counselor is finished, the authorized connection to the central database is closed. In a system with comprehensive data security, an audit trail, indicating the time, date, data requested, and identity of the counselor, would be recorded on the central database system.

Client/Server Computing

Client/server computing indicates a functional relationship between two computer systems. The "client" is typically a user with a computer, connected to the network, who needs to interact with data resources stored on one or more "server" databases located elsewhere on the network. Servers also provide other services to their clients, including access to centrally located, shared resources such as printers, scanners, faxes, archival storage, and shared hard disk storage. Servers may also provide clients with access to other network resources such as the Internet over a shared network linkage to an Internet service provider (ISP).

In the client/server model, the client computer shares some of the work load of a given task with the server. Many clinical information systems use this model. A client program, which is installed on the user computer, is responsible for the "look and feel" of the clinical information system. The client program handles queries and data input from the user and negotiates data transactions with the server database transparently to the end user. The client then displays the information and may additionally provide data analytic functions such as statistical analysis, graphing, or print reports. In some cases, depending on the nature of the query, statistical or other calculations based on stored data may be performed by the server and the results forwarded to the client. Whenever processing is done on the client, the work load of the server is reduced, allowing it to serve more users. This must be balanced with the volume of data that must be transferred to the client for the necessary analysis to be done. Queries that access large amounts of data can overwhelm the network and degrade performance for all users—and may be better accomplished as a server based task.

The chief drawback to the client/server model is the installation, configuration, and updating of the client software on all clients. In a large network, several hundred client workstations in different geographic locations may need to be configured and updated as new releases of the client software become available. This can be an enormous task, especially when the client computers are different brands, running different operating systems. When the client computers include a mixture of Intel/IBM compatible systems, Apple computer products, or Unix workstations, the complexity increases significantly. Assuming client software is available for each class of computer system to be used (by no means assured), the installation and configuration of the client software can be very different for each, requiring distinct skill sets on the part of the installer.

In large networked environments, where client-computing resources can be standardized, it is possible to install software management clients on all systems, which allows for centralized distribution of software upgrades to all clients. This eliminates the need to travel to each computer and individually install software. This type of management client (which can even upgrade itself) is commercially available and can dramatically reduce the cost of supporting client systems.

The Web Browser as Universal Client

The explosive growth of the Internet and World Wide Web as well as the proliferation of intranets (restricted access networks that provide internal services to a defined group or organization) has made the Web browser the standard interface of choice for many applications. Any computer, regardless of processor type or operating system, equipped with an Internet compatible browser can connect to, and interact with, any Web server. As long as all interactions between the browser and Web server are conducted using Internet standards [e.g., HTML (Hypertext Markup Language), FTP (File Transfer Protocol), Java, XML (Extensible Markup Language), etc.] supported by both systems, the Web browser/server model can provide the same access to resources that the client server model does. One significant advantage is that the client computer only needs to be "Internet ready." All of the work of accessing and processing data as well as controlling the layout of the user's screen (i.e., the "look and feel" of displayed information) is shifted to the server side in this model. The only exception to this is the ability of the browser to download and run "applets" from the server. Applets are typically small Java- or Active-X–based programs that are executed by the browser and provide application-specific resources or utilities to the user. An applet might perform calculations on retrieved data and plot a graph, or facilitate the construction of a complex query to be submitted to the server. Applets can pose potential security problems, since they involve executing programs accepted from a remote computer. It is possible for a rogue applet to cause damage either by erasing or stealing confidential data, or as a means of propagating a computer virus. It is important for the end user to be able to trust and verify the source of the applet to be downloaded and executed. Authentication strategies, including digital certificates and trusted authorities that validate certificates by digital countersignature, reviewed in the section on encryption, below, can provide a means to verify the source of an applet before it is downloaded. Browsers such as Netscape Navigator and Microsoft's Internet Explorer have configurable security options that can selectively restrict or prohibit Active-X– or Java-based applets. While disabling applets entirely provides a high degree of security, it may also interfere with trusted Web-based applications that use applets. Another option is to configure browser software to accept only applets that are accompanied by certificates signed by a trusted authority. A list of trusted authorities can be specified in the browser security options.

Databases and Database Management Systems

There are two distinct topological classes of database systems: central and distributed. Each class has distinct advantages and disadvantages. Hybrid models, which incorporate elements of both classes, offer many advantages but are more costly. In the central database design, all data are stored on a single, typically large, computer. The centralized system allows fast cross-sectional access to all data. Physical security is simplified and all access to the data can be controlled from a single, centralized authentication process. There are several important liabilities in the centralized design: there is no redundancy; if the system goes down, all data is inaccessible; and any breach of security potentially exposes the entire database. There are ways of compensating for these weaknesses, such as disk mirroring, which involves redundant parallel writing of all data transactions to a second "mirror" disk that can be switched to in the case of primary disk storage failure. A complete mirror computer system running in parallel with the primary system safeguards against catastrophic system failure but essentially doubles the cost.

The distributed database model offers many advantages in behavioral health information systems. In this model, data components are stored on multiple computer systems that serve specific functions but are networked together. In the case of a hospital, each department, core administrative function, or clinical service might have its own clinical database with data unique to its function. Another example would be a behavioral health system with multiple clinics, each with a local patient database, linked together over a leased network connection. In the distributed model, patient data are stored on multiple computers. Billing and demographic data are stored on one system, while medications and allergies are stored on another. Consequently, the aggregate patient record exists only as a virtual construct or "view" that must be assembled by querying the respective component databases. This assembly should be carried out by the clinical information system and be transparent to the end user.

The advantages of distributed database systems include local control and management of data as well as some degree of fault tolerance. If one system goes down, the others may still be able to function. For example, in the case of the networked mental health clinics, if one clinic server failed, it would still be possible to access patient data for all patients except those whose data was stored on the failed system. Disadvantages of the distributed model include more complex information system administration, and increased risk of security breaches due to multiple systems at different locations. Potentially the most significant problem is that of data synchronization, that is, ensuring that redundant data components stored in different locations are updated at the same time. For example, core demographic data are frequently stored redundantly in several different systems, such as, in the case of a large clinic, patient registration, pharmacy, and laboratory systems. When patients' demographic data change due to address change, marriage, etc., it is critical that these changes are implemented in all locations. One approach to synchronization is the inclusion of time stamps on data fields, that is, additional data fields that store the date and time that each database field was entered or updated. A simple protocol can then be implemented to ensure that the correct and most current information is replicated.

Hybrid database models incorporate design elements from both the central and distributed database designs. While by design, these systems incorporate redundancy of data storage, they do not merely duplicate function, as in the case of the "mirror computer system." One realization of the hybrid model is a combination of a distributed database system with a central data repository or "warehouse." In this model, the warehouse contains a copy of some or all of the data stored on the distributed systems. The warehouse data are updated whenever corresponding data at a distributed site are changed, ensuring synchronization. The warehouse thus serves as an on-line backup and can be configured to provide data whenever a distributed component fails or is off-line. The warehouse provides an efficient resource for cross-sectional searches and data analysis (on-line analytical processing). Cross-sectional searches across the distributed database system are much more inefficient since multiple queries need to be issued and then assembled. These queries also degrade the performance of the distributed system for the primary clinical users.

The choice of database design is driven by several considerations. The size and complexity of the behavioral health entity will dictate the computational requirements of the information system. For example, a small private practice with a single clinician and a receptionist serving a few to several hundred current patients (including the capacity to store inactive patients for up to 5 years) would be adequately served by a shared-access database system running on a modest personal computer as a "central server" and linked by an office network to one or more "client" personal computers.

Regardless of the central or distributed nature of the database management system, its chief functions are the storage, retrieval, and analysis of data. Several layers of software may be interposed between the physical (electronic) storage and retrieval process and the ultimate display of clinical information on a computer screen or in a printed report. Security issues and implementation of confidentiality policies, discussed below, must be considered at all levels, from the physical location of the computers to operating system, database management system, and clinical information system software. Security and data protection capabilities need to be included from the earliest point in the design of systems and software. It is difficult or impossible in most cases to retrofit secure data management capabilities onto preexisting software.

While operating systems and clinical information system software are discussed elsewhere in this book, it should be noted that even as new and comprehensive clinical information systems are becoming commercially available, there has been a rapid increase in the complexity and diversity of data types that must be accommodated. These newer data types include digitized radiographic images, pictures, electrocardiograms (ECGs), dictated voice data, and video. Some of these data sources are in digital format from the point of acquisition, such as computed tomography (CT) and magnetic resonance imaging (MRI) scans. Others, such as ECGs, scanned documents, voice dictation, and video, may be acquired in analog or digital format depending on the technology used (e.g., digital video camera versus analog VHS video camera), and may need to be preprocessed into digital format prior to storage. One example of the rapid growth of newer data types is the use of video conferencing technology for remote consultations. So-called telepsychiatry consultations, where the clinician and patient are in different locations and connected by a high-speed video and audio connection, are becoming more common, especially in specialized environments such as prison systems and geographically remote and underserved areas of the country. These video sessions can be integrated into the medical record in a variety of ways, including digital storage in a large-capacity database system.

Networking, Communications, and Data Interchange

Most large behavioral healthcare clinical information systems consist of a patchwork of legacy systems coexisting with clinical software applications and are also linked to core clinic/hospital information systems such as the pharmacy, laboratory, radiology, etc. Clinical data may be stored in databases located on departmental servers and may be replicated in enterprise-wide data repositories or "data warehouses." The ease with which these data are accessed and integrated into functional views of aggregate and individual patient data depends critically on the structure and format of the data and on the ability of the respective software systems to communicate with each other. This communication can take several forms. The least sophisticated method of data interchange between two information systems involves a data export function on the part of the sending system and a data import function on the part of the receiving system. The computers do not even need to be physically connected. Data can be exported to magnetic disk or tape or optical media and physically transported. If the systems are part of a network, then this exchange can be accomplished on-line, assuming both systems can read and write to a common location. More sophisticated, "real-time" data interchange can take place if both database management systems support a standard query language such as SQL. An SQL query that specifies the requested data would be generated by the requesting system and sent over the network to the database management system, which stores the required data. Assuming the requesting party has authenticated itself properly (e.g., with username and password), the responding database management system would return an electronic message containing the data requested. Depending on the security protocols in place, this entire transaction may be encrypted to prevent eavesdropping or interception of data as the data travel over the network.

A critical and often problematic part of this data exchange between two clinical database systems is the identification of corresponding data elements. For example, one database system may store patient gender using a field called "sex," indicated by a numeric code where 1 corresponds to male and 2 to female. Another data system may store a "gender" field that uses character data "M" and "F" to designate this. A database that has hundreds or thousands of data elements per patient record may differ significantly in the format and coding of stored data. Each pair of communicating systems therefore requires a "translation table" to match corresponding data elements and to convert from one coding/data format to another. In a large distributed computing environment, such as a hospital or integrated delivery system with several to hundreds of computer systems from different vendors running different operating systems and using specialized applications software, the work required to implement the necessary translation software for N different applications or systems increases as $T = N*(N - 1)/2$, where T is the number of translation programs that need to be created. This problem can be greatly reduced, so that only $T = N$ translation programs are necessary by adopting an intermediate standardized data format for all data to be imported from and exported to. The problem is then reduced to writing translation software for import/export to this standard format for the N systems. Products that facilitate this process are sometimes referred to as "universal interface" products.

There has been considerable effort to develop standards for the interchange of health data between different computer and software systems. One proposed national messaging standard is HL 7 (www.HL7.org). Standard vocabularies for health information data are also being developed that would define the name and format of all health data elements in the medical record. If a standard vocabulary were to be adopted, the problem of identifying corresponding elements between clinical databases would be greatly simplified. Currently there are several proposed standard vocabularies and hundreds of different code sets [such as ICD-9-CM, ICD-10 (International Classifications of Diseases), SNOMED (Systematized Nomenclature of Medicine), CPT (Current Procedural terminology), etc.], prompting the development of meta-vocabulary software that could serve as a "thesaurus" between standard vocabularies.[1]

Health Insurance Portability and Accountability Act

In 1996, Congress passed the Health Insurance Portability and Accountability Act (HIPAA).[2] The bill, sponsored by Senators Edward M. Kennedy and Nancy Kassebaum, was intended to protect insurability when workers changed jobs. The act mandated Congress to pass legislation on health information privacy by August 21, 1999. The act further directed the secretary of the Department of Health and Human Services (DHSS) to implement a policy on health information privacy by regulation in the event that Congress failed to meet this deadline. Congress did not meet its self-imposed deadline, leaving Secretary Donna Shalala of DHSS with the mandate to promulgate regulations to protect the privacy of health information. Specifically, HIPAA requires the creation of standards for the storage, security, and communication of health information. It also requires the creation of a unique identifier for each individual, employer, health plan, and healthcare provider in the United States.

Preliminary information on the forthcoming regulations has been published in the Federal Register by the secretary of DHSS as "Notices of Proposed Rule Making" (NRPM) and is available on the Web (http://aspe.hhs.gov/admnsimp). Several NRPM documents have been published outlining proposed regulations for the unique national provider and employer identifiers, security standards, and health information privacy. Due to significant controversy and objection by many national organizations including the American Medical Association and the American Psychiatric Association,[3] legislation was passed by Congress, placing further work on implementing a unique individual identifier on indefinite hold.

On August 17, 2000 the secretary of DHSS published "Health Insurance Reform: Standards for Electronic Transactions" in the Federal Register.[4] Standards including data format and code sets are established for eight electronic health insurance transactions that transmit individually identifiable healthcare information including healthcare claims, healthcare claims status, coordination of benefits, health plan premiums, eligibility, enrollments and disenrollments, healthcare payment and remittance, and referral certification and authorization.

All healthcare providers, healthcare insurers, and healthcare data clearinghouses that use electronic transactions will be required to comply with the regulations following a 2-year implementation period. Small health plans will have 3 years to comply. Those electing to use paper transactions would not be affected by the regulations.

The goal in creating uniform standards for data format, content, and security for healthcare-related electronic transactions was to increase the efficiency of the process and lower administrative costs, which account for a disproportionately large portion of healthcare-related expenditures.

The Protection of Electronic Behavioral Health Information

An understanding of the importance of privacy in the healthcare provider–patient relationship dates back to the time of Hippocrates. Since that time, physicians, swearing the Hippocratic oath, have promised to keep their patients personal health and other information confidential, considering such knowledge, obtained in the practice of their art, and elsewhere, as "sacred as secrets."[5]

The advent of computerized clinical information systems has simultaneously provided the means to enhance the quality and coordination of services offered by a healthcare provider and the means to breach confidentiality on a scale unprecedented in the history of the traditional paper chart. In the absence of effective security measures, it is possible to search for and extract sensitive data on, for example, human immunodeficiency virus (HIV) status or history of past suicide attempts, on hundreds or thousands of patients in a matter of seconds or minutes.

Such breaches have already occurred. In 1996, an anonymous person sent a list of almost 4,000 HIV persons in Florida's Pinellas County to the Pinellas

County Health Department and to two newspapers. The sender claimed the list came from a Pinellas public health worker who mislaid it in a gay bar.[6] A Pinellas County Health Department worker who allegedly used the data to screen dates was later charged.[7]

The goal of implementing effective security policy and technology for a behavioral health clinical information system is to prevent unauthorized access to confidential data without impeding that use by authorized individuals. This is most effectively accomplished when security and confidentiality concerns are addressed as the clinical information system software is being developed. It is very difficult, if not impossible, to retrofit data security features onto an existing application.

Physical Security of Health Information

The physical security of the computer hardware including peripheral devices such as external hard drives as well as removable disks and archival media of all types is of paramount importance. Data may be accessed from an unprotected computer in a variety of ways: the hard disk may be removed and its contents probed using another system, or the computer may be forced to "boot up" (start up) from a floppy disk, bypassing various software protections, and the database file simply copied, searched, modified, or destroyed.

All computers containing patient data, from data center machine rooms to individual servers, should be in locked, restricted areas. Where this is not possible, such as small offices without a separate computer room, it is possible to physically lock the chassis of the computer and securely attach it using commercially available mounting plates to a desk or counter. It is also desirable to physically lock access to any bootable disk drives using keyed disk-size inserts, or to easily disable system startup from any floppy or removable media device using the computer's (BIOS) setup configuration utility. This prevents unauthorized users from starting the computer using different operating system software, bypassing the installed operating system and application specific security features that would be functional if the system was started normally.

A physical security consideration frequently overlooked is the data stored on computer systems and storage media that are resold or discarded. Unless properly erased or destroyed, confidential data can be recovered from even damaged computer disk drives. Disaster recovery software, commercially available, can be used to recover data from computer disks that have been erased or even reformatted using nondestructive erase or format utilities. For example, a used computer sold to a computer consultant in Nevada contained information on 2,000 customers of a supermarket-based pharmacy chain in Tempe, Arizona. The data included patient names, social security numbers, as well as medication lists. The list identified individuals taking medications including Antabuse, azidothymidine (AZT), as well as a variety of psychiatric medications.

Failed fixed storage devices such as hard disk drives are subject to potential data recovery unless they are physically destroyed. Functional computers, storage devices, and reusable storage media should be destructively erased using commercially available software utilities that overwrite all data (multiple times), preventing future recovery. In some systems, a destructive erase capability is included as part of the basic operating system utilities. Non-reusable data storage media such as CD-R disks and other "write once" optical media must be disposed of in a secure manner that ensures physical destruction.

Firewalls and Network Security

Firewalls are an important first line of defense for any internal network or even single computer connected to the Internet or other external network. Even though behavioral health clinical information systems typically have several layers of security implemented at the clinical application, database management system, and operating system levels, a firewall can defeat many attempts at unauthorized access at the earliest point possible. A firewall's chief function is to protect an internal network from unauthorized access from the external network. It can also be used to restrict some or all external network access by internal users. A firewall is typically a dedicated computer running specialized firewall software. It should be the only computer that has a direct connection to an external network. Its task is to monitor and filter according to customizable criteria, all incoming and outgoing network data packets. Firewall security software can be configured with rules that are specific to individuals or groups of users. Any network activity including e-mail, FTP (file transfer protocol), Telnet, and World Wide Web access can be regulated by the firewall. For example, the firewall may be configured to allow incoming or outgoing email, but refuse all Telnet (remote login) connections unless the user is authenticated by a valid firewall account (user ID and password). Firewall software is also commercially available to protect from unauthorized access home or small office computers that are used to connect to the Internet. Home or office computers with full-time Internet access, running operating systems that allow sharing of peripherals, and hard disk storage devices are at significantly higher risk of unauthorized access via the Internet than dial-up users with intermittent network connections.

Encryption

Although encryption technology offers the means of significantly increasing the security of health data, its use in health care is not widespread. Encryption offers the ability to encode clinical databases so that only authorized users can retrieve decoded data. If the database is accessed by an unauthorized user bypassing the clinical information system, perhaps using a database utility program or a low-level hard disk inspection utility, the contents of the database would be unreadable. Data communications over networks including the Internet can be encoded so that eavesdroppers cannot access the data being transmitted. Virtual private networking is accomplished by sending encrypted data packets over public networks, which offer a cost-effective alternative to private leased network connections. Video conferencing and telemedical audio/video transmissions and recordings for consultation or healthcare delivery can be encoded either in digital or analog format using commercially available products. Archival data, including disaster recovery data, that are stored in remote locations may be encrypted to prevent unauthorized access. Data may be encrypted multiple times. For example, disaster recovery tapes that contain a backup copy of a clinical database that is already encrypted may be encrypted a second time during the backup process since it may be stored at a remote, possibly less secure location. Two (or more) separate password keys would then be required to decode any clinical data from the archive.

Higher levels of security as well as functional partitions of databases can be achieved by differential encryption of clinical data. A clinical database in a large hospital information system might store information on hundreds of thousands of patients. It is possible to implement an encryption process that encodes each patient record with a different key. Furthermore, demographic data, primary care data, infectious disease data, and psychiatric data may all be encoded differently if desired. Note that restricted and differential access to clinical data in a role-appropriate fashion is more a function of the design and function of the clinical information system than of the encryption used, but the use of differential encryption does make it possible to afford particularly sensitive data a higher level of protection. In the case of differentially encrypted records, the computational complexity of accessing multiple patient records by unauthorized means (i.e., "cracking" the code) increases dramatically. The prospects of breaking the code on even a single record is poor. Data protected by password keys of sufficient length (1,024 bits or longer) using the current public key cryptography would require millions of years of time using the fastest, most powerful supercomputers currently available.[8] As computers become more powerful, it will be necessary to use longer key lengths. There is also the very real possibility of advances in number theory that may lead to new approaches to factoring very large numbers. Such an advance could render an encryption standard obsolete and would require implementation of a new encryption method.

Encryption does not protect against fraudulent use of valid access codes stolen from an authorized user. The use of encryption also increases the amount of computational work associated with storage or retrieval of data. Consequently, the choice of an encryption algorithm for a clinical information system is, to some extent, a balance of security needs and system performance. Fortunately, the evolution of computer technology continues to follow Moore's law: computing power doubles approximately every 18 months. The use of encryption also creates a new problem: the management and security of the password keys that are needed to lock and unlock data, which must be handled by the security functions of the clinical information system.

The most familiar form of encryption is symmetric or secret key encryption. Data to be encrypted are combined mathematically with a password key to generate a random-appearing string of coded data. To successfully decode the data requires that the coded data be combined mathematically with the password key.

The Date Encryption Standard (DES)[9] is the U.S. and international standard for symmetric data encryption that uses a 56-bit key. Programs that implement DES are widely available. The DES standard is now dated due to the rapid increases in computer technology and government restrictions on the length of the key. DES-encoded data can now be broken in a matter of days (or less) using a specialized code-breaking computer or supercomputer and is due to be replaced by the Advanced Encryption Standard (AES) by the National Institute of Standards and Technology (NIST). Variants of DES, such as Triple DES, which uses a 112-bit key, remain extremely secure although computationally more expensive.[10]

Symmetric encryption can be used to encrypt data communications or email messages but a fundamental problem exists. For the message to be decoded by recipients, the key must be known to them. How can the password key be securely transmitted to recipients? This is essentially the problem of sending a secure message in the first place. An elegant solution to this problem is the public key encryption algorithm.

Public Key Encryption

Public key algorithms form the basis of secure communications, digital signatures, and digital certificates that can be used to authenticate received digital signatures. Public key encryption algorithms are asymmetric. That is, different but related password keys are used to encrypt and decrypt. One key of the key pair is called the public key; the other is the private key. A message encrypted with one key can only be decrypted with the other key from the pair. Key pairs are unique; given one key it is mathematically possible, but computationally extremely difficult, to calculate the other key. The computational difficulty increases with longer key length. Longer keys, therefore, offer increased protection.

In the public key model, users keep their private key secret but publish their public key widely. Anyone who wishes to send a message to these users needs only to obtain their public key and use it to encrypt the message. Only the holder of the private key can decrypt the message. Using this method, the sender can also electronically "sign" the message before sending it. Suppose Bob wishes to send Mary a confidential report. Bob first "signs" the message by encrypting the message using his private key. At this point anyone possessing Bob's public key would be able to decrypt and read the message, and would know that it came from Bob. Bob then obtains Mary's public key and uses it to encrypt the signed message. This ensures that only Mary will be able to read the message and she will be able to verify that the message came from Bob since the message was signed with his private key. One weak link in this system is if Bob does not keep his private key private, allowing someone else to impersonate Bob by using his private key. Figure 2.1 illustrates the encryption–decryption process using public key encryption.

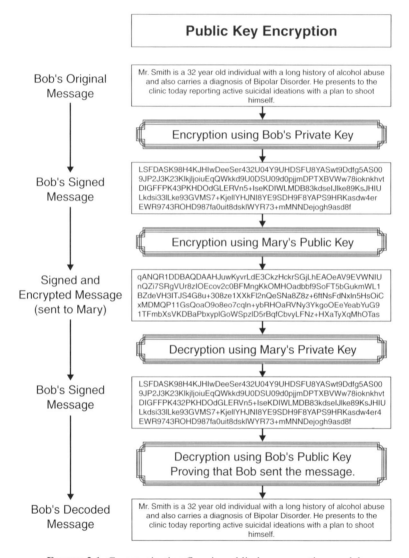

FIGURE 2.1. Communication flow in public key encryption model.

The next level of security involves certificates. If someone publishes a public key claiming to be a certain individual, how can this be verified? In the above example of Bob and Mary, suppose that a third party, Beth, wished to intercept the confidential report. Beth could do this by placing her own public key where Mary's should be. Bob unknowingly uses Beth's public key to encrypt the report that would then be readable only by Beth. Having intercepted the message and read it, Beth might also then encrypt Bob's signed message with Mary's true public key and forward it to her, pretending to be Bob. This is an example of a "man in the middle" attack. Beth could continue to intercept messages going both ways with neither Bob nor Mary knowing that their messages were being read.

Certificates and Digital Signatures

How can Mary's public key be verified as actually belonging to Mary? It could be verified if Mary had registered with a trusted authority or certification authority (CA). The trusted authority is responsible for verifying the identity of an individual and creates a digital certificate containing the registered individual's public key and name signed with the authority's own private key. Anyone wishing to send Mary a secure message would use the CA's public key to extract Mary's public key and name, which verifies Mary's public key, and then use her public key as described earlier. Obviously, this process only works if the CA is trusted. Digital certificates also include an expiration date. A number of commercial entities offer CA services. Businesses, hospitals, universities, and other organizations can use commercially available software to set up CA services for their own information systems.

Public key encryption is an ideal method for secure communications. The only complication is that it can be difficult to find someone's public key. Currently there are no widely implemented standards for the required public key infrastructure. A public key infrastructure would standardize the storage and network (e.g. Internet) access of public keys, and provide a directory or search function that would enable a user to find an individual or business public key regardless of where it was stored.

Any behavioral health entity wishing to use public key encryption to secure data and communications can set up a local public key exchange system using commercially available software. As standards for public key infrastructures and key exchange evolve and are implemented widely, the basis for secure, verifiable communication with other healthcare providers, healthcare insurers, and patients (who will have their own verifiable certificates) will be established.

User Authentication

The best security and encryption technology in the world is powerless to prevent unauthorized access by someone who has stolen legitimate access codes from an authorized user and who has physical or network access to the information system. As discussed, the traditional user ID/password pair is very insecure. Many individuals in a behavioral healthcare setting access multiple computer systems requiring different user ID/password pairs. It is very common to find these user ID/password pairs written on paper taped to the wall or even on the computer monitor where they are easily visible to others.

The security of the information system can be significantly increased by implementing authentication technology to help verify the identity of users at the time they attempt to access the system. Authentication technology can augment or, in some cases, replace the user ID/password pair.

Something You Have and Something You Know

This technique combines the user ID/password pair with a portable technological token that must be presented to the system along with the user ID/password. One example of this technology, currently commercially available, is a key fob–sized device that has a liquid crystal display that shows a number that changes every 60 seconds or every few minutes. This number is synchronized with a corresponding device integrated with the clinical information system security. An authorized user must present both a user ID/password pair and the current number displayed on the device in order to be authenticated by the system. Any unauthorized user who wanted to gain access to the system would now have to obtain a valid user ID/password pair and steal the authorized user's key fob device. Other authentication technologies, based on smart cards (credit card–sized devices that contain data storage and microprocessor technology) are also available and can provide authentication using cryptographic techniques. These typically require a smart-card port to be installed on the computer to be used to access the system.

Biometrics

Potentially the most stringent level of authentication, biometric authentication, involves the scanning of some unique physical characteristic such as a fingerprint, iris shape, retinal blood vessel pattern, infrared facial characteristics, hand geometry, and voice print. These patterns are compared against a security database containing the known biometric patterns for all authorized users. Some biometric authentication systems measure two or more biometric characteristics to increase accuracy and decrease false-negative rejection rates (instances where the authentication process fails to recognize a valid user).

The use of biometric authentication requires that a sensor be attached to the computer system. Sensor costs range from approximately $100 for a fingerprint sensor to over $1,000 for a retinal scanner with complex optics. Fingerprint sensors are now available integrated into a PC card that can be used to secure access to a laptop computer or other computer equipped with PC card ports. Fingerprint detection, currently the most cost-effective and widely available biometric technology, has a high degree of reliability, and is acceptable to most users, but can potentially be circumvented.[11]

Policy and Legislative Issues

Health information will never be adequately protected until comprehensive federal legislation is passed. Privacy protections under forthcoming HIPAA regulations based on the published Privacy NRPM (Notice of Proposed Rule Making)[12] are considered by many to be inadequate and apply only to the electronic records of healthcare providers, insurers, and data clearinghouses. The American Psychiatric Association, among others, criticized the proposed privacy regulations as actually lowering privacy protections.[13] In her proposed recommendations to Congress in 1997, as required by HIPAA, Secretary Donna Shalala of DHHS called for Congress to pass comprehensive privacy legislation protecting health information. As of October 2000, Congress has failed to pass privacy legislation. State laws offer varying degrees of protection of health information.

Local policies, which govern the security and confidentiality of health information data, are also critically important. Every individual who is authorized to access patient information must be informed of the institutional policies and state and federal laws and regulations regarding the protection of health information.

Whenever possible, clinical information systems should be implemented so that healthcare workers can access only information necessary for their appointed role. Role-specific views of clinical data have been implemented in many clinical information systems. For example, a nurse must be able to access medication and laboratory data on a patient but would not normally need to access outpatient psychotherapy records. Audit trails that document which patient records were reviewed, and by whom, should be implemented and reviewed regularly by a designated security manager. Automated reports can be generated based on certain types of user actions. For example, any user who accesses an unusually large number of patient records or a record designated as "VIP" can trigger a special audit flag. It is imperative that policies are enforced as well as published. Sanctions proportionate to the breach of confidentiality, up to and including dismissal, should be clearly stated in the confidentiality policy manual.

References

1. Tang PC, Hammond WE. A progress report on computer-based patient records in the United States. In: Dick RS, Steen EB, Detmer DE, eds. *The Computer-Based Patient Record: An Essential Technology for Health Care.* Washington, DC: National Academy Press, 1997.
2. Health Insurance Portability and Accountability Act of 1996, Pub. Law No. 104-191; enacted August 21, 1996.
3. *Psychiatric News* 1999;34(2).
4. Department of Health and Human Services, Office of the Secretary, Health Care Financing Administration. Electronic transactions: announcement of designated standard maintenance organizations: final rule and notice. *Federal Register* 2000;65(160). (Available on the Web at http://aspe.hhs.gov/admnsimp.)
5. Bulger RJ. 1987. The search for a new ideal. In: Bulger RJ, ed. *In Search of the Modern Hippocrates.* Iowa City, IA: University of Iowa Press, 1987:9–21.

6. AIDS Policy Law, 1996 Oct 18, 11:19, 11.
7. *Houston Chronicle,* February 15, 1997, p. 15A.
8. Schneier B. Key length. In: *Applied Cryptography: Protocols, Algorithms and Source Code in C.* New York: Wiley,
9. *American National Standard for Data Encryption Algorithm (DEA).* ANSI X3.92. Washington, DC: American National Standards Institute, 1981.
10. Kaufman C, Perlman R, Speciner M. Data encryption standard (DES). In: *Network Security: PRIVATE Communications in a PUBLIC World.* Englewood Cliffs, NJ: Prentice Hall PTR, 1995.
11. O'Gorman L. Fingerprint verification. In: *Biometrics: Personal Identification in Networked Society.* Norwell, MA: Kluwer Academic, 1999:43–64.
12. *Federal Register* 2000 V65 #250 Pg 82461–82510. Department of Health & Human Services "Standards for Privacy of Individually Identifiable Health Information".
13. "APA Fighting Accord for Better Medical-Record Privacy Rights" December 3, 1999. *Psychiatric News* 1999;34(22):1.
14. National Resource Council. *For the Record: Protecting Electronic Health Information.* Washington, DC: National Academy Press, 1997.

Part II
Clinicians' Issues

Introduction

ROSS D. MARTIN

Welcome to a brave new world. Our technology revolution has continued to rage along with unprecedented acceleration to the point that—like a jet bursting through the sound barrier—we have moved ahead far faster than our ability to consider all the implications of our advances. The combination of ever-cheaper, ever-faster processing power and ever-broader, ever-expanding networking capabilities has given us new opportunities to impact the human condition right where it can impact our quality of life most—our mental health.

Using computers in the behavioral health arena is nothing new; in fact, one of the first clinical applications utilizing minicomputers involved the collection of psychiatric histories.[1] Since those early efforts, the Internet and its accompanying connectivity technologies have enabled clinicians to aggregate and disseminate just-in-time information as never before. Some applications, such as educational programs and data collection tools, are a current reality. Others, such as real-time decision support, are relatively new additions to the clinician's toolbox and must still survive the rigors of our academic and peer-reviewed process in the literature before they are fully embraced. Still others are only now being imagined and researched.

Time will tell if the summation of the "telecom's" impact on the human psyche ultimately does more harm than good. My personal suspicion is the latter, though no doubt the relatively isolating nature of our current use of technology will provide a ready stream of patients seeking relief and understanding from the behavioral health provider community. But use it we must.

The chapters in this section offer a glimpse of some of the directions we are heading in behavioral health informatics. Read the findings, predictions, warnings, and conclusions of the authors. Then consider them all again in a dozen years to see how closely our brave new world resembles their forecast. Whatever the outcome, it promises to be a very interesting ride.

Reference

1. Maultsby MC, Slack WV. A computer-based psychiatry history system. *Arch Gen Psychiatry* 1971;25:570–572.

3
Knowledge Delivery and Behavioral Healthcare Professionals

ROBERT KENNEDY

Health care is the largest information business in the United States economy. One third of its trillion-dollar cost is the cost of creating and processing information.[1] The general lack of standards makes it difficult, expensive, and time-consuming to establish the simplest forms of communications. If it is difficult for patients to get a second opinion or to compare outcomes data for different institutions or procedures, imagine how difficult it is for a clinician to scan the qualifications of specialists in order to make a referral. This chapter discusses the science, history, and trends related to information and knowledge sharing and how technology will transform the behavioral health "knowledge worker" for years to come.

A Brief History of the Knowledge- and Information-Seeking Person's Need to Connect to Others and Exchange Information

In the world of behavioral health, the smallest basic unit of information is the neuron. Why start here? This is where it all began and why we study behavioral health. It is fascinating to observe that there is a prime directive for connection at the cellular level. Neurons share a common organization dictated by their function, which is to receive, process, and transmit information.[2]

In human development, the single cell information processor, the neuron, seeks connections to other neurons. It branches to bundles and ultimately stretches to increased levels of specialization. It develops sophisticated channels of communication from presynaptic levels of "preprocessing" to postsynaptic "data dialogues" that give our nervous systems extremely complex and rapid methods of handling information. All of this results in a complex data system that can effectively process local information and handle the complexity of incoming data with relative ease.

As we mature into a sophisticated information processing system, the prime directive remains the same as that of the single neuron—to receive, process, and transmit information. These processes give us the ability to process, and interact with, the environment. These are the basics of communication and shared knowledge. Knowledge acquisition requires interaction and connections. Our survival as a single entity depends on this communication system.

In interacting with the environment, we generally seek connections to, stimulation from, and contact with other individuals and groups of people. We also seek the products resulting from the thinking and creative output of others; these are the rewards of collaboration. In our brain's multiplicity of connections, the more we use a connection the easier and more facile it becomes.

To some extent, our survival as a civilization has been dependent on our ability to communicate, cooperate, and collaborate with others, and combine resources and effort. So too in our assessment of computer development, the smallest unit, the transistor, which comprises the microprocessor, by design seeks connections to other components to perform its functions. There is increasing sophistication, for example, graphic processors and coprocessors, and these "electronic synapses" connect to each other and share the computing responsibilities. Since we have begun using computers for many complicated but mundane tasks, we have been connecting them to other computers to share information. These connections form the backbone of business, education, and information systems, and they continue the process of sharing human information that began with the neuron.

With the advent of computer networks, the workplace has also become a shared computer environment. There are local and wide area networks as well as virtual private networks that are active in work groups sharing projects or video conferencing. Thus, with the Internet and the World Wide Web, the global connection has begun.

There is now an enhanced merger of the computer with the human connection. Humans have evolved their connections to each other, encompassing other cultures and races without regard to geography. Over the centuries, as people traveled the earth, the distances became smaller and the connections between people strengthened. The global computer network has now connected millions of people who may never have traveled or connected in any other way. The world has become smaller and more accessible.

Early Knowledge Delivery Vehicles

This need to convey knowledge led our ancestors to seek consistent ways to communicate information. They began with the verbal tradition. Stories that described various life events served as poignant messengers of knowledge. Learned behaviors derived from either observation or from listening to the stories of adventurers or elders who had ventured beyond one's immediate world were used for coping with many of the difficult situations in life. Thus, knowledge was recognized as a precious commodity early on. Information about herbal treatments for illness and other early medical procedures were verbally transmitted from one generation to the next within families or from a master, such as a shaman to an apprentice. These masters were the first behavioral healthcare specialists and were revered for their knowledge.

Our continued mission to communicate and connect presented itself as our next challenge. How do we record and transmit knowledge? Some of the first writings on stone, and later papyrus, were used to document transactions between people, tell stories, and educate. With the advent of writing came the ability to convey information over a greater distance and carry the original message through many generations. To transmit recorded information to other scholars during the Middle Ages, manuscripts were painstakingly copied by hand until Gutenberg devised a method to duplicate information in a fraction of the time. The dissemination of information, which had been an important function for all civilizations, could now be done through printed material. Legal and medical texts became some of the most important textbooks.

Knowledge Delivery Today

To make healthcare and behavioral healthcare information available, the more traditional and popular forms of information sources (books, journals, monographs, letters to the editor, newsletters, etc.) are being supplanted by on-line versions that are easier to access and have capabilities that their paper counterparts do not. They can be searched across multiple volumes, quickly accommodate requests for articles by a specific author, and link to Medline abstracts or other forms of information. Many on-line versions offer the abstract of an article, and others provide the full text.

Most traditional journals have an on-line counterpart. While some offer free access, many charge a subscription fee. Other types of information offered by professional Web sites include journal reviews that summarize salient articles in the leading journals, drug information, and specialty or general health news. This is an evolutionary period for print journals, and the advantages of the Internet (speed, ease of use, new ways of combining information) present new challenges for traditional publishers. Continuing along the evolutionary pathway, many of the newer journals are E-journals only. The process from review to publication has been dramatically shortened thanks to the ease and speed of on-line publishing.

Since the Internet is a democracy, anyone can publish anything. Search engines can find everything from a sophisticated book chapter to crude hate mail. Thus, the message is, "Reader beware." When we access information, we need to consider the sources. It is worth taking a few moments to check the integrity of a Web site: Who runs it? Who owns it? What editorial procedures are used? Are the posted articles written by healthcare professionals or credentialed medical writers? Is there an editorial board? Are the articles peer reviewed? These are some of the questions that one should be asking about information on the Net, especially healthcare and behavioral healthcare information.

Since the Net is such a pliable medium and offers many ways of presenting information, it makes sense that we would try to adapt many types of knowledge acquisition to fit this platform. In addition to traditional books and journals, there are other methods of learning that healthcare professionals consider beneficial to their development, such as conferences and meetings of the professional organizations and associations in various disciplines. Rooted in tradition, these well-attended specialty meetings are where colleagues exchange ideas, learn from one another, and update their training with continuing education (CE) or continuing medical education (CME) courses. These too are being translated into the domain of the on-line world. Conference reports, treatment updates, symposia, and review courses are transcribed and made available to professionals who either are unable to attend a conference or missed a particular session and wish to learn about what was presented.

Knowledge and Information Dissected

We have a complex relationship with knowledge, especially clinical information. We gather facts into discrete units and then combine them or compile them into impressions. The discrete unit is initially important but remains so only if we attribute weight (value) to it; the importance of the discrete unit depends on its degree of impact on the impression or whether or not it has impact on other aspects of clinical work.

For example, obtaining information in an interview about a patient's sleeping patterns or habits might reveal a sleep problem, such as insomnia. This problem may be a result of increased alcohol intake or a symptom of an anxiety disorder. It may also be secondary to a physical problem (asthma or gastroesophageal reflux). The sleep problem may ultimately result in poor job performance, irritability, and difficulties in interpersonal relationships.

Learning to use diagnostic decision trees or following treatment algorithms has offered tremendous benefit to the clinician. Decision trees are an organized and structured way to gather and understand clinical data. The treatment algorithms present a structured systematic guideline for assistance in making treatment decisions.

How is it possible to translate clinical information into knowledge that can be an on-line resource? To take this challenge one more step, how can we get on-line clinical information at the point of care? Understanding what information is important in a simplified model is easy. Clinicians know what information they need to do a competent job. However, this model becomes quite complex as we realize the speed of change in clinical information. We now have to deal with the latest treatment approaches, the newest pharmacological interventions, and the most recent research findings as they are made available. Integrating constantly updated information into a current knowledge base can be an information-processing nightmare.

To help solve this dilemma, we need to revisit the concept of weighing information. Publishers of on-line articles must "tag" important elements of the article and prioritize them for rapid retrieval, perhaps even at the point of care. Authors and editors need to tag important aspects of the presented clinical information and create a link that can be retrieved, indexed, and synthesized quickly.

For example, a psychiatrist is working with a patient who has a treatment-resistant depression. At the point of care, while reviewing the on-line electronic medical record, he can log on to a clinical Web site that has just published an article by an author he respects on the latest review of treatment-resistant depression. Since time is of the essence in this situation, he just wants the highlights. His query offers two possible treatment approaches: (1) a medication that recent studies have found to be effective, or (2) cognitive-behavioral therapy to supplement the patient's current medication. The psychiatrist makes a decision feeling confident that he has embarked on a better treatment plan for the patient. If he has more time, either before or after seeing the patient, he can review a Medline abstract or read the full article offering strategies for handling the difficult-to-treat depressive disorders. He can also review the evidence-based material on the success of various treatments.

This line of sophisticated questioning requires a new understanding of the value of knowledge and information and that publishers and authors plan ahead to allow subsets of the information to be utilized. They also need to ensure the integrity of the information, present the information in context, and verify that it communicates sound clinical data.

Knowledge Acquisition

The challenge to past and future civilizations has been and will be the pursuit of knowledge, and specifically how to acquire it, how to use it, how to store it, and how to disseminate it.

Knowledge acquisition accompanies curiosity. Seeking information on many different levels adds complexity both to our quest for and to our use of information. For example, a therapist doing group therapy needs to understand not only each of the individuals in the group, but also the group process, which is a separate entity. In addition, he needs to be aware of the discussion's impact on the process as well as on each individual in the group. This layering of information creates a complex interaction and a challenge to even the most skilled therapist. The point is that information or knowledge rarely stands alone. So many characteristics or qualifiers, some more important than others, need to be considered.

Medical students who learn patient interviewing in a psychiatry clerkship often want to jump to a diagnosis in the first five minutes. They have not yet learned that every clinical encounter cannot be condensed into a one-line diagnosis, and have not yet appreciated how the details can help in understanding the patient. In their desire to quickly understand and fix the presenting problem, they often overlook salient points and subtleties of behavior that a more sophisticated interviewer would not miss. To address this problem, a new approach is being used to teach students to gather and integrate information more effectively. Case-based teaching offers a broader view of patients in the context of the various systems in which they function.[7]

Direct Knowledge Acquisition

The traditional method for the exchange of information since the time of the early shaman or of the Greeks and Romans has been the mentoring or supervisory relationship. Trade apprenticeships, such as physician mentoring, enable the student or apprentice to learn the necessary skills and methods for performing procedures in their particular trade. This is still an important method of direct exchange of information today. It ensures the quality and integrity of the information. The supervisory or mentoring relationship has been considered the pinnacle of training in many fields, and communicating knowledge by supervision and first-hand experience has been the basic premise of medical training.

Other methods of information exchange include classroom instruction, association meetings, and conferences. Students take CME or CE courses to obtain the specialized knowledge that is difficult to obtain elsewhere. This method, relatively unchanged from its early Greco-Roman roots, is the academic standard for communicating knowledge by direct exchange, often supplemented with books or manuscripts. In specialty conferences, leaders in a particular field offer words of wisdom to the participants.

Indirect Knowledge Acquisition

Indirect methods of gathering knowledge include books, journals, manuscripts, and letters. These utilize the written approach to disseminating information and offer a well-organized way to present information. The advantages of this method of exchange are that it is replicates readily, reaches a great number of people, and is easily transported great distances. Medical school is a prime example of when the indirect method combines with the direct, because books supplement classes and supervised lab or clinical experiences.

Knowledge Acquisition Today

Today we take information from traditional forms and recombine it in new ways. We build on our historic methods of knowledge exchange and enhance them with new technologies. Although the classroom remains an important place to learn from the masters, today the classroom extends beyond its walls through recording techniques, interactive teleconferencing, and other technical enhancements. The concept of a "university without walls" can now have a global reach.

We can also combine information in new ways to change learning. We can change views or perspectives on information instantly by using computer technology. For example, in a discussion of epidemiology, a lecturer can display a graph and instantly change data elements for "what-if" scenarios. This lecture can also be transmitted simultaneously into a remote lecture hall, to individual networked computers, or across the globe. Interactive video conferencing and telemedicine have a similar global range.

People can interact in a variety of ways, not only with a mentor but also with each other. Much as students gather after class to discuss what they have learned and share insights with each other, we can enhance this learning process via technology. E-mail, chat technology, list servers, and other forms of electronic communication offer ways of augmenting knowledge acquisition without the limitations of time or place. Thus, teachers can interact with students in a group or on a one-to-one basis.

The ability to supplement information has also changed dramatically. In a traditional school setting, a student seeks reference material in a library. Today, information can be gathered in class, at home, or anywhere else with a computer connection. In a less direct fashion, courses can be set up for self-instruction via computer, so that individuals can learn at their own pace and at a time they choose.

Internet and the World Wide Web

The Internet will affect knowledge exchange through its multimedia and hypertext capabilities. The Internet is easy to use, has global reach, and lends itself to standardization.

By 2005, it is expected that a billion people will have access to the Internet. By 2010, Web-enabled appliances are expected to outsell personal computers by a factor of 10 to 1.

Standardization

What makes all of this connectivity possible was the establishment of standards. When the Internet was established, part of the wisdom that allowed for its universal adoption is a set of standards or protocols [Transmission Control Protocol/Internet Protocol (TCP/IP)] that established a simple and relatively inexpensive global communication system.

Hypertext, Multimedia, Nonlinear Learning

Part of the magic of the World Wide Web is its inherent style of interaction. Hypertext (meaning "beyond text") links allow movement or "jumps" to other pages of related information and to other Web sites regardless of location.

When we read a page in a book, we may come across a word that we find interesting or unusual. We stop reading, think about the word and how it is used in this context or in another context, and perhaps even look it up in a dictionary. After this digression, we go back to the page and resume reading. That is how hypertext works. It allows for interaction with knowledge in a way that is more analogous to the way we think. We can jump to a hypertext link (digress) or follow a logical sequence and interact easily with multimedia elements to enhance learning. This changes the way we acquire knowledge and the way we interact with information. By design, a Web page allows many types of media, including text, pictures, sound, video, and animation. These are also the elements of multimedia, and they enhance our interaction with knowledge in ways that are closer to the way we naturally learn.

Nonlinear Learning

Nonlinearity offers a learning style and interaction with information that is more natural and emulates the way we interact with the world. Nonlinear interaction allows the person to explore information from any point. Unlike a book, which has a beginning, middle, and end, a nonlinear approach offers the opportunity to start in the middle or anywhere else to explore information. Hypertext allows for this approach and offers new opportunities for learning and interaction.

Technology Versus Knowledge

Marshall McLuhan[4] advocated that we not be blinded by technology. But today we are enamored of technology. Because the computerization of information is still in its infancy, we amuse ourselves by attempting to obtain the fastest computer processor or the largest color monitor available on the market. We often forget that the whole point of technology is to lead us to the information, and then accumulate and process it for us. In some ways, it is akin to driving a car. After we learn to use the vehicle, we no longer think about the process of driving. It becomes an automatic process and we focus instead on where the machine will take us. We need to focus on the tasks of learning and interacting with knowledge, not on the technology itself.

We are often impressed with the dazzle of special graphics on a Web site or an elegant design of an instructional CR-ROM. But other than demonstrating an imaginative interface, does it assist us in gathering information? This brings to mind a clever cartoon showing a person standing in front of a colorful and ornate Web page. The caption read: "This is great but where is the door?" Designing with the transfer of information in mind is still uncharted territory. The interface should not impede or complicate the acquisition of knowledge. Learning should be a clearly marked road; we need to be able to navigate ourselves to the information we want quickly and easily. Presenting information in a palatable and friendly way is more difficult than it sounds. A tremendous amount of planning and testing goes into creating an interface that is simple to use and easy to navigate. It is quite difficult to make something look easy.

Technology can either enhance or interfere with knowledge acquisition. We need to encourage colleagues and trainees to develop educational programs, algorithms, guidelines, clinical reference tools, and study materials. We also need to encourage them to follow the principles of good design in the creation of these programs.[3] One must always remember that the goal is to *inform* and *educate* rather than impress or dazzle the reader.

Technology can facilitate knowledge in many ways. The concept of "always-on" connections is spreading from the university and business world to the home computer with high-speed connections. This creates vast possibilities for information exchange. Individuals can now make their personal libraries available for searches, catalogues, and data engines. For example, suppose that Dr. Smith spent a year researching panic disorder in adolescents or that Dr. Jones did her dissertation on posttraumatic stress disorder (PTSD). With appropriate security measures, they can make their research notes, reference lists, and background material available on-line. This can save other clinicians and scholars innumerable hours of replicating the same work. In turn, others can share new information or findings with Drs. Smith and Jones to enhance their own knowledge bases.

As various technologies merge, such as local or mobile personal networks and wide-area networks, their corresponding information appliances (Internet-ready cell phones, hand-held computers) proliferate; any information can be available from anywhere at any time.

Bertrand Russell said, "Language serves not only to express thoughts, but to make possible thoughts which could not exist without it." He believed that unique and novel ideas and forms of expression were born from new combinations of familiar elements. The World Wide Web has given us opportunities to interact with knowledge and thus has expanded our abilities and created a unique subset of communications that may not have been possible otherwise.

Empowering Ourselves Before Empowering Others

Part of empowering ourselves through knowledge is learning about available tools that help us understand data. If we rely on the information management staff to tell us what information we can obtain and how we can view it, we are doomed to a dependency that will leave us somewhat helpless and only partially informed.

We must learn to use the tools that we need to manipulate the data ourselves. This is the only way to have adequate control over the data. If we wish to evaluate a particular data set and look at its impact on other variables, or run a "what if" scenario, we can easily learn to accomplish this. For example, if the staff in a psychiatric emergency room (ER) is recording demographic and clinical data into a database, a number of "canned" reports can then be generated. But staff members who know how to question and manipulate the data have power over the data and can create their own queries, such as, How many females between the ages of 18 and 25 have come to this ER with a presenting problem of suicidal ideation and no previous history of depression? They can then change one variable in the query and acquire new information: On which days is the ER visited heavily? Which shift gets the most patients? Staffing patterns can then be adjusted to optimize the resources in the ER and put manpower where it is needed most.

To obtain empowerment over the data, we must gain an understanding of the data set that we are using, and learn what fields are used to collect information. Then we will know what is being collected and what information can be extracted. We also must learn to use the tools that will assist us in directly manipulating the data. If we are not using the tools ourselves, we must understand their power and capability so we know what questions to ask. Otherwise we must rely on someone else's judgment about what we might need or want.

The tools range from the simple database or spreadsheet to the more complex statistical package. Any of the popular databases or spreadsheets can import or export data and offer the tools needed to query, view, or graph data in a variety of ways. The learning curve is the approximate couple of hours spent learning the interface. With a statistical package, the learning curve is steeper and is generally for the student serious about data or those interested in research.

Evidence-Based Clinical Information

One of the goals of sharing knowledge is to learn from the accumulated wisdom of others. In clinical practice, standards are established for the various assessments, therapeutic approaches, and treatments. Keeping current with the latest clinical and scientific findings in the field of mental health is a formidable task. A method is needed to synthesize information and evaluate the best scientifically verified treatments, as there are numerous treatments for the same disorders. This is the domain of *Evidenced-based Practice* (EBP). In a serious attempt to narrow the gap between research and practice, clinical practice is being influenced by EBP guidelines and clinical reviews as seen at the Cochrane Library[5] (Mulrow, 1994) by utilizing the tools from clinical epidemiology, biostatistics, and information science. EBP is derived from evidence-based medicine. According to Sackett et al,[6] "Evidence-based medicine is the conscientious, explicit and judicious use of current best evidence in making decisions about the care of individual patients. The practice of evidence-based medicine means integrating individual clinical expertise with the best available external clinical evidence from systematic research."

The American Psychiatric Association publishes the *Diagnostic and Statistical Manual of Mental Disorders* in an attempt to encourage the use of a more scientifically rigorous set of diagnostic criteria derived from well-documented clinical research. The use of these standardized criteria also facilitates a wealth of research that was not previously viable. In the last two decades, we have accumulated an unprecedented amount of epidemiological, genetic, neuroanatomical, and clinical data. This work led to the recent interest in using EBP in the mental health field. One of the fundamental tenets of EBP is that specific study designs are best able to provide unbiased answers for different types of clinical questions. For example, good-quality randomized trials (either single trials or meta-analyses of several comparable trials) for treatment produce the most valid estimates of a treatment's effectiveness.

The information and knowledge needs of the behavioral healthcare professional include the following: patient data, such as history, mental status, testing, and physical findings including laboratory data, x-ray, diagnostic imaging, and special tests; field reports from the ER, hospital, caseworkers, ACT (Assertive Community Treatment) teams, home health workers, urgent care centers, caregivers, and employers; treatment plans; and general information such as behavioral health and medical knowledge and research; medical, psychiatric, and behavioral health news; medication information; patient education information for dispensing to patients; referral information; and insurance information. These are very complex data needs that require a great deal of integration and coordination of information. A true challenge for this decade is getting all of this information in one place for clinicians so that they may be well informed and make good treatment decisions. Solutions such as the enhanced electronic medical record can offer ways to manage and negotiate the complexities of these informational needs.

The information and knowledge needs of the patient/consumer include the following: laboratory data, X-ray, diagnostic testing results; hospital, ER, and field reports; medication information; consultant reports; educational materials; behavioral health and medical knowledge and research; medical, psychiatric, and behavioral health news; referral information; and insurance information. Patients will gain increased access to their clinical information and participate in clinical decisions and treatments.

What to Expect

In the late 1400s, Leonardo DaVinci conceived airplanes, helicopters, and parachutes—all as sketches in his notebooks. It took centuries for these concepts to come to fruition because in DaVinci's time the distance between what his mind could imagine and what technology could deliver was immense. Today, our technological capabilities are much more sophisticated. However, with our need for immediacy we become similarly frustrated, because what we imagine—continuous speech technology and software that acts on our behalf—might take a few years to become a viable reality. So, what does the future have in store? The primary issues that will drive progress will be communication and information, not processing power. Of course, e-commerce will facilitate progress; it will also open pathways to information and communication that would have been otherwise unaffordable.

We are currently in the early, accumulation phase of information gathering. This is much like starting a library, where the first phase is obtaining books and journals. We are acquiring and storing information of every imaginable type—from sports stadium seating plans to world news that changes hourly. The goal is to make this information available 24 hours a day to anyone who wishes access to it.

The second phase of information acquisition is organizing the material in a way that provides easy access. The on-line world has been described as the "Library of Congress with no card catalogue." To search or index effectively, we will require not only clever software but also a set of standards for cataloging all of this knowledge.

The third phase is to let the information work on our behalf. In addition to sophisticated indexing of information, we need to give information catalogues the ability to "think for themselves." Such catalogues will be able to act independently and solve problems or recombine information in ways that were not previously possible.

We can now concentrate on more sophisticated software programs that can assist us in the gathering and organization of our information.

Electronic Medical Record (EMR)

The EMR or Digital Health Record (DHR) as it is also called on-line health record will become an essential part of the delivery of health care. It offers capabilities far beyond the paper record including:

• Ease of access to charts (rapid retrieval)
• Organization and legibility (consistently well organized and readable)
• Flexible data entry tools (pop-ups for fields to minimize typing)
• Real-time decision support (alerts, reminders)
• Work-flow automation (fewer steps than paper, e.g., for a prescription refill)
• Population-based reporting (can send physician letters/email about clinical alerts or drug recalls)
• Connection to hand-held or wireless devices.

The EMR will also make available clinical encounter support tools such as previsit questionnaires and assessments as well as postvisit information and support.

Agents

Intelligent-assistant programs such as software agents, can carry out our instructions and perform a number of tasks on the Internet. These small software programs can automate a number of tasks and carry out "informational" interactions on our behalf. For example, after giving the agent a set of directives, it can traverse the Internet, do a Medline search, check to see if a particular book is available to purchase as well as its cost, and order flowers for a friend's birthday using our credit card and electronic signature. It finally returns to give us a status report of its activity.

As these programs become more sophisticated, they will be able to carry out a complex set of instructions that will provide us with calendar reminders and database searches. They will organize data and write a preliminary report for us after learning our particular preferences and style.

Collaboration

Discourse with colleagues will always be a priority in health care. The use of electronic media will broaden the channels of interaction and allow for communication in novel ways. On-line case consultations, supervisory sessions, virtual conferences, and grand rounds will become as commonplace as e-mail and list

TABLE 3.1. Provider-based needs for digital knowledge.

Give me most of the information that I want and all of the information that I need
Give it to me as fast as I need it (speed of thought)
Make it available to me anywhere at anytime.
Offer me multiple graphic views of the information so I can quickly grasp the complexity and the impact
Suggest directions for using this information based on a history of my preferences (remember my style)
Let me pull salient facts quickly and recombine them into a comprehensible package (combination of word process, grammar check, reference check)
Let me send it to whomever I wish or to another computer for a different perspective on my data
Track the processes, time, interactions, quality, and outcome measures; report relevant answers to me quickly and complete reports as needed.

servers. The ability to be in two places at once is one of the dramatic advantages of such connections. Distance is irrelevant. If, for example, you live in New York City and you wish to attend grand rounds at Stanford University, you could either be a click away from a live presentation or replay an archived version at a more convenient time. Collaboration via the Internet has also extended the office into the home and changed the way we traditionally think about education and interaction with colleagues.[8] The grand rounds can also be interactive (whether live or archived), where the Web participant can ask questions or participate in discussions via video cam, e-mail, or discussion forum. Greater degrees of information are available in a variety of ways.

Healthcare Web sites have proliferated for both professionals and consumers and will continue to play an important role in the sharing of information. Access will be available in a variety of ways, from standard computer interfaces to handheld devices to Internet appliances (Table 3.1).

References

1. Boston Consulting Group, "Managing for a Wired Health Care Industry", INVIVO, July/August 1996.
2. Yudofsky S, Hales R. *Textbook of Neuropsychiatry.* 3rd ed. Washington, DC: American Psychiatric Press, 1997:4.
3. Black R. *Desktop Design Power.* Washington, DC: Bantam Electronic Publishing, 1991.
4. McLuhan M. Understanding Media. New York: McGraw-Hill, 1964.
5. Mulrow CD. Rationale for systemic reviews. *BMJ* 1994;309:597–9.
6. Sackett DL, Rosenberg WM, Gray JA, Haynes RB, Richardson WS. Evidence based medicine: what it is and what it isn't. *BMJ* 1996;13[312(7023)]:71–72.
7. Albanese MA, Mitchell S. Problem-based learning: a review of literature on its outcomes and implementation issues. *Acad Med* 1993;68:52–81.
8. Kramer T, Kennedy R. Educational computing: the World Wide Web and Internet: online communication, collaboration, and collegiality. *Acad Psychiatry* 1998;22:66–69.

4
Decision Support Tools in Psychotherapy and Behavioral Health Care

Lawrence G. Weiss

The informatics revolution in behavioral health care opens the door to data-based therapy management using real-time clinical decision support tools. In most settings, however, the application of an empirically based continuous quality improvement approach to clinical care is far from the reality. Clinical decision support tools are the keys to unlocking this potential.

Clinical decision support tools are a broad class of procedures designed to support behavioral healthcare providers with information as they make important decisions about patient care. In a sense, this is not a new idea. We have had decision support tools from the very first computer-generated interpretive reports for the Minnesota Multiphasic Personality Inventory (MMPI),[1] although we did not initially use that terminology. Many of today's tools go much further in recommending specific courses of action, such as level of care determinations, recommendations about types of therapy or treatment techniques that may be most efficacious for a given disorder or set of patient characteristics, patient readiness to step down in the continuum of care to a less restrictive and less expensive setting, and recommendations for discharge or termination of outpatient treatment. With so much at stake in terms of patient welfare, as well as the economics of providing behavioral healthcare services, it is important to critically evaluate these tools. This chapter reviews four major areas of concern in evaluating clinical decision support tools: research quality; implementation issues; ethical and practice issues; and cost, both direct and indirect. A discussion of the five types of decision support tools is also reviewed.

Evaluating Decision

In evaluating decision support tools, the foremost concern is the integrity of the research. What is the quality of the research that upholds decision support algorithms? Some systems utilize predictive algorithms based on 30 years of academic research, while others are developed from individual experiences with a single beneficiary population. The research documentation may be buried in internal corporate technical reports, or worse yet, validated on college students.

The quality of the questionnaire that resulted in these algorithms must also be considered. Many technical psychometric issues need to be considered when developing outcome instruments for use with decision support tools. Outcome measures typically require different psychometric characteristics from those required by traditional intake assessments. Outcome measures must be sensitive to clinical change, whereas intake instruments must adequately discriminate between diagnostic groups with high rates of sensitivity and specificity. These diverse purposes of discrimination and sensitivity to change have a dramatic effect on the types of items selected during the test construction process. Items on intake instruments must cover the primary disorders with sufficient depth to reliably distinguish between them. Items on outcome measures are more often selected to measure changes in symptoms or functional status and must be state-based rather than trait-based in order to detect improvements during treatment. All of these reliability and validity studies should be conducted on appropriate populations, with adequate statistical controls, and should be published in peer-reviewed journals or other sources open to professionals qualified to judge the adequacy of the data.

The major factors effecting successful implementation of a decision support system in clinical practice are the "fit-with-work" flow and the usefulness of the information to the clinician. If technology requires an interruption in the routine flow of work, or if it requires an additional step not otherwise performed, the clinical staff will be less likely to use the technology itself. When the rate of participation drops below a certain level, the data are called into question. Compliance will improve if information is fed back to clinicians in a timely manner and if that information is viewed as helpful. Systems in which data are collected locally, mailed or faxed to a remote location for processing, and then returned to the clinical site on a monthly or quarterly basis are likely to suffer from noncompliance. If managerial pressures are applied to improve compliance, such as making payments for services contingent upon receipt of all required questionnaires, then compliance may improve, but the quality and accuracy of the information may be poor due to the misplaced incentive. Systems that provide meaningful clinical information in real time are inclined to achieve the highest compliance rates with implementation.

Regarding ethical practice, the main issues involve the qualifications of the person utilizing the decision support tool, and the organization's view of the decision support information as prescriptive versus descriptive. As these tools become more automated, some organizations place them in the hands of less qualified caregivers who may not be clinically qualified to make independent decisions about patient care. They may rely too heavily on the output of the machine, failing to consider extenuating circumstances when it is appropriate to do so.

As market forces push prices even lower, this purely technological practice without human intervention is possible. That is, the output of the tool is viewed as the decision, rather than as information that supports the clinician as he or she makes the ultimate decisions about patient care. Such views tend to obscure the need for qualified clinicians to evaluate the information in the context of the full clinical picture.

Long-term and indirect costs must be balanced against short-term direct costs. Most organizations will consider the cost of the materials or the service as well as the cost of the clinician's time. One trap to avoid is planning for the staff to enter data that have been aggregated at a central location. For example, one large hospital chain required that all clinicians batch and send their outcomes measure to a central location, and then discovered it needed to hire a full-time employee to key in hundreds of questionnaires per day. Although centralization may entail certain economies of scale, it does not allow true decision support to occur at the site of care.

One possible solution is to computerize the local practitioner's office. While technology can be costly, the costs need to be evaluated in relation to the costs of hiring key-entry operators to enter data collected on paper combined with the cost of licensing paper versions of copyrighted assessments. Providers who are responsible for population-based issues and are under capitation arrangements tend to take a systemwide perspective and balance these short-term direct costs against the cost of making an incorrect clinical decision, or the cost savings from reducing relapse rates and medical offset due to improved care. These cost-offset studies are urgently needed.

There are many different approaches to decision support, and the relative advantages and disadvantages of each can be judged with respect to research quality, implementation issues, ethical practice issues, and the ratio of direct costs to indirect cost offsets. There are at least five broad classes of decision support instruments available on the market today. These are matching diagnosis with goals, matching patient and therapist characteristics to treatment techniques, the use of longer but more psychometrically sophisticated instruments, automated treatment formularies, and the modeling of recovery curve trajectories.

The first method involves matching diagnostic problems to specific treatment goals. This approach takes a problem orientation and seeks to link specific presenting problems to observable and measurable goals. With practice management software, it becomes possible to track progress of these goals and to graphically view client progress plotted against important clinical variables such as number of sessions, type of therapy, and type of medication. At the individual level, the practitioner can see the effects of changing medications or adding group or couples therapy on the client's goal attainment, and use this information in making decisions about continuing, changing, or terminating a particular clinical path. At the aggregate level, one can observe trends in the number of sessions required to successfully treat specific diagnostically related problems and use this information for establishing treatment guidelines and clinical protocols used to support and guide clinical decisions in the future.

This approach is usually easy to implement and presents few ethical practice problems because it is consistent with how clinicians typically think about these problems. It is also consistent with the movement of various regulatory agencies toward problem-oriented medical records. Because this approach simply tracks progress on goals linked to problems, there is little need for a strong research base. The issues that support the logic in the software application need to be addressed, however, once the aggregate information is used to develop guidelines for clinical care.

The second class of decision support tools involves matching patient characteristics to particular therapeutic techniques or levels of care. Here, the clinician assesses critical patient variables, such as degree of reactance, coping style, extraversion versus introversion, motivational distress, and the degree to which the presenting problems are complex and thematic versus simple and symptomatic. Depending on the patient's relative standing on each of these variables, he or she may be more or less likely to respond to different treatment approaches. For example, a patient who is low in reactance and extroverted and has no complex symptoms may benefit from a directive approach like cognitive behavioral therapies that focus on particular external behaviors. On the other hand, patients who are highly reactant, introverted, and thematic may respond well to less directive forms of treatment involving an insight orientation or focusing on interpersonal dynamics. Levels of motivational distress indicate the extent to which the therapist should employ supportive techniques versus other techniques designed to arouse the client. This approach is most associated with Larry Beutler at the University of California, Santa Barbara.[2]

The body of research supporting this approach is quite large and of good quality. This type of patient-to-treatment matching may be difficult to implement because of the need to collect considerable patient information on each of these variables. Practice issues abound in locating therapists skilled at each of the recommended techniques and ensuring that they are properly trained and are correctly implementing the techniques. However, the clinical division of the American Psychological Association is moving toward promoting and disseminating manuals about empirically validated therapies for specific disorders to therapists, thus possibly providing a solution to the training dilemma.

An example of an approach that seeks to match patient characteristics to level of care (LOC) decisions is the Severity and Acuity of Psychiatric Illness Scales developed by John Lyons[3] at Chicago's Northwestern University. This method involves staff rating of several critical variables including suicide risk, danger to others, severity of symptoms, difficulty with self-care, substance abuse, medical complications, family disruption, vocational impairment, residential instability, motivation for treatment, medication compliance, knowledge of illness, family involvement, and persistence of symptoms. These variables are used in decision support algorithms to predict the probability of a risk-appropriate inpatient admission versus one that is risk inappropriate. Once again, the quality of the research data is good, and while there may be implementation issues with interrater reliability across shifts or across staff professions, it is hard to say that these variables are unimportant to LOC decisions.

Another category of decision support tools involves the use of longer, but more psychometrically elegant, instruments. There is considerable literature on treatment planning with the MMPI, for example, as well as many other traditional clinical instruments. Systematically assessing patient characteristics known to facilitate or impede the treatment process can be very helpful in predicting and controlling length of stay or the number of outpatient sessions. For example, closed-mindedness, low expectation of therapeutic benefit, lack of social support, problems in relationship formation, and self-absorption are all variables that research has shown to have impact on the course of treatment. Individuals who are closed-minded and self-absorbed, for example, will likely be difficult cases requiring higher levels of clinical supervision, more intensive case reviews, and a greater number of sessions to work through these hindrances in order to treat the presenting symptoms. This approach is evident in the Butcher Treatment Planning Inventory, which measures patient characteristics and correlates them with treatment process issues.[4]

The quality of the research supporting these types of assessments is consistent with a long history of psychometrically sophisticated instrumentation with good reliability and validity. Proper use of the information would seem to raise the bar for clinical practice. While some practitioners may not be aware of methods for working with patients who present with these types of roadblocks, the early identification of these issues, combined with effective clinical supervision, may prevent futile sessions where significant behavioral healthcare resources are utilized but no clinical progress is made.

Another class of decision support tools involves comparing automated reviews of treatment plans against an electronic treatment formulary. Here, the organization's treatment formulary is programmed into algorithms in a central server. Providers' treatment plans are sent electronically to the managed care organization where the plans are run against the formulary. If there is a positive match with the formulary, an authorization is returned electronically to the provider, or more information is requested. If the plans are inconsistent with the formulary, they are automatically assigned to a live case manager for review. This approach is taking shape with a number of software applications, including one called OPTAIO, by the Psychological Corporation.[5]

The major advantage of this approach is in the implementation. Care requests are approved more rapidly, with fewer case managers, and with assurances that authorizations are consistent with approved formularies. Those responsible for creating the formularies at each of the managed care organizations are also responsible for the quality of the literature reviews, thus largely impacting the research quality. Ethical practice issues are of real concern, however, in that some organizations may seek to automate denials of care without live reviews. It is essential that in these cases knowledgeable case managers evaluate the exceptions and extenuating circumstances with good judgment of clinical input. A few practitioners may also "learn the ropes" and fashion their requests in ways that would gain automated approval. Such gaming is, of course, unethical and is a potential problem any time strict treatment guidelines are implemented.

The final class of decision support tools under discussion here is the type that seeks to monitor patient progress and rate the clinical significance of the patient's improvement against some standard. The work of Neil Jacobsen and Paula Truax[6] of Washington University leads the field in conceptualizing this approach. Traditional outcome studies have looked only at the statistical significance of the change between pretest and posttest scores. However, with large sample sizes, even very small changes in mean scores can be statistically significant. This is why the current draft versions of the Standards for Psychological and Educational Testing strongly encourage researchers to move away from a rigid reliance on statistical significance and place more emphasis on effect sizes. In other words, assuming the finding is significant, the subsequent question is, What is the size of the effect? In the arena of outcomes research, Jacobsen and Truax have taught clinicians to ask, How clinically meaningful is this outcome? They propose a series of possible methods for answering this question based on the relative probability that the posttest score is more likely to be drawn from the normal distribution or the clinical distribution. These methods have been adapted and computerized for the Beck Depression Inventory,[7] Devereux Scales of Mental Disorders,[8] and several others. Clearly, knowledge that a particular patient's progress in treatment can be reliably assessed as "positive but insufficient" or "very favorable" provides the clinician and case manager with objective information. The information can be used to support clinical decisions about continued authorizations of treatment, stepping down in the continuum of care, or termination of treatment.

This approach is strongly based in quality research data. Implementation issues may surface initially with the need to have patients tested repeatedly, but provider resistance can be mitigated by the availability of useful clinical feedback in real time. Cost is also an issue with repeated testing, but is now being made affordable through paperless administrations. Studies that evaluate these direct costs, as compared to the potential long-term indirect cost savings from reducing relapse rates and lengths of stay, as well as medical offset studies need to be conducted.

However, this approach does not stop here. The field is going further in monitoring patient progress, rating the clinical significance of the patient's improvement against some standard direction, and attempting to model patient recovery trajectories. Also called "dose–response curves," this system is most associated with Ken Howard et al[9] of Northwestern University in Chicago, and with Michael Lambert and Gary Burlingame and colleagues[10] at Salt Lake City's Brigham Young University. Here, a standardized assessment, such as the Outcomes Questionnaire–45, is administered repeatedly to a large group of patients during the course of treatment and an average recovery curve is developed. The availability of an average recovery curve in real time allows providers to track the progress of individual patients against this trajectory during the course of treatment.

There are some very difficult statistical issues inherent in this approach. Perhaps the most important is the issue of risk adjustments to the data. If the recovery curves are to be differentiated by diagnosis—still an open question—it is quite clear that not all patients with the same diagnosis can be expected to make progress at the same rate. Consider two patients with major depressive disorder. One is 35 years old, in his first episode of care, employed as a manager in McDonald's for 10 years, and in an unsatisfactory second marriage of 5 years. The other is an unemployed, divorced 24-year-old, in her third episode of care with a *Diagnostic and Statistical Manual of Mental Disorders*, 4th edition (DSM-

IV) Axis II diagnosis of borderline personality disorder, two potentially lethal suicide attempts in the past 6 months, and a history of mixed substance abuse. Although the major diagnosis is the same, the goals, treatment plans, and expectations for these two patients will be very different. Recovery curves must therefore be risk adjusted based on some measure of the complexity of the case, independent of diagnosis.

An assessment of case complexity should include variables that previous research has shown to be important in psychotherapy outcome research. These include variables such as perceived lack of social support, highest previous level of functioning, consistency of previous functioning, expectations of therapeutic benefit, agreement with current treatment plan, history of compliance with medication regimen, evidence of Axis II personality disorders, medical complications, substance abuse, danger to self or others, and more. All these data considerations need to be taken into account when either designing or examining computer-based decision support systems for psychotherapy.

In conclusion, it is worrisome that computers may make important decisions about patient care, especially if these tools are viewed as justification for hiring providers with less training and education. These individuals will be less able to recognize the inevitable situations when the decision support algorithms are inconsistent with the clinical realities. In addition, if they do happen to recognize them, they are less secure in their independent judgments and more likely to defer to the perceived expertise of the computer. At the very least, a live case manager should routinely review any automated denial of care decision.

The definition of clinical decision support tools offered earlier was worded very carefully to address these concerns and it bears repeating. Clinical decision support tools are a broad class of procedures designed to support clinicians with information as they make important decisions about patient care. It does not say that clinical decision support tools "automate decisions about patient care based on expert logic programmed into a piece of software." There are those who say that these tools should produce only narrative reports about what has been found helpful based on peer reviewed research, thus providing information that supports the decision making process without actually *making* the decision. But are these tools intended to be prescriptive or descriptive? Ultimately, the culture of the organization that implements the tool will determine the manner in which it is used. In an organization that has a strong clinical culture with effective clinical supervision, these tools can be an asset to both practitioners and managers of behavioral healthcare services. Real-time clinical decision support tools can assist the organization in achieving the goal of consistency in practice settings based on the best empirical evidence.

References

American Educational Research Association, American Psychological Assocation and National Council on Measurement in Education. *Standards for Educational and Psychological Testing*. Washington, DC: Author, 1999.

1. Hathaway SR, McKinley JC. *The Minnesota Multiphasic Personality Inventory Manual*. New York: The Psychological Corporation, 1951.
2. Beutler LE, Berren MR. *Integrative Assessment of Adult Personality*. New York: Guilford, 1995.
3. Lyons JS. *The Severity and Acuity of Psychiatric Illness Scales: Manual*. San Antonio, TX: The Psychological Corporation, 1998.
4. Butcher JN. *Butcher Treatment Planning Inventory: Manual*. San Antonio, TX: The Psychological Corporation, 1998.
5. The Psychological Corporation. *OPTAIO Practice Manager* (version 2.3.0) [computer software]. San Antonio, TX: Author, 2000.
6. Jacobsen NS, Truax P. Clinical significance: a statistical approach to defining meaningful change in psychotherapy research. *J Consult Clin Psychol* 1991;59(1):12–19.
7. Beck AT, Steer RA, Brown GK. *Beck Depression Inventory Manual*. 2nd ed. San Antonio, TX: The Psychological Corporation, 1996.
8. Naglieri JA, LeBuffe PA, Pfeiffer SI. *Devereax Scales of Mental Disorders: Manual*. San Antonio, TX: The Psychological Corporation, 1994.
9. Howard KI, Lueger RJ, Martinovich Z, Lutz W. The cost-effectiveness of psychotherapy: dose-response and phase models. In: Miller NE, Magruder KM, eds. *Cost-Effectiveness of Psychotherapy: A Guide for Practitioners, Researchers, and Policymakers*. New York: Oxford University Press, 1999:143–152.
10. Lambert MJ, Hansen NB, Umpress V, et al. *Administration and Scoring Manual for the OQ–45.2*. Stevenson, MD: American Professional Credentialing Services, 1996.

5
Computerized Medication Algorithms in Behavioral Health Care

Madhukar H. Trivedi, Janet K. Kern, Tracy M. Voegtle, Shannon M. Baker, Kenneth Z. Altshuler

Advancements in medicine have occurred rapidly over the last several decades. These advances have taken place in areas such as basic medical knowledge, treatment strategies, interpretation of clinical data, diagnostics, and pharmacology, thus changing the extent and complexity of medical practice. Physicians in clinical practice (specialists as well as primary care physicians) are called upon to assimilate a substantial volume of complex data for a multitude of medical conditions. Physicians' decisions in clinical practice not only are contingent on a considerable knowledge base, but also require the physician to stay well informed of current advancements in order to optimally treat patients.

In an effort to facilitate this process, various tools have been designed to manage the large amounts of new information and keep everyday medical practice in sync with current technology. Guidelines are among the methods most frequently used for this purpose. In study settings, the use of clinical practice guidelines and algorithms has been shown to be effective in assisting doctors in clinical decision making, thereby improving clinical practice.[1–23] However, in routine practice, guidelines and algorithms are significantly underutilized, primarily due to limits in their immediate availability and ease of use at the time of patient care.[4,24–29]

Medical technology is making considerable progress in the design and utilization of computerized medication algorithms to support clinical practice. Computer-assisted clinical decision support systems (CDSSs) have the potential to overcome many of the limitations of paper-and-pencil clinical guidelines and algorithms.[30,31] The availability of CDSSs has focused considerable interest in the usefulness, applicability, and rich potential of these computerized tools in assisting with patient care.

This chapter gives a brief history and description of clinical guidelines and algorithms, and discusses the uses and advantages of computerized medication algorithms as decision support systems, particularly in behavioral health care. Factors that can inhibit optimal implementation of these tools, and recommendations for improving the usefulness and practical applicability of CDSSs are discussed. Important considerations concerning software design are also addressed. Finally, the computerized treatment algorithm (CTA) in development at the University of Texas (UT) Southwestern Medical Center is described in its current stage.

Clinical Practice Guidelines

Clinical practice guidelines (CPGs) were first introduced in the 1960s for the management of emergency medical situations. They have since been developed for a number of medical disciplines, and continue to grow in popularity and diversity. Defined as "systematically developed statements to assist practitioner and patient decisions about appropriate health care for specific clinical circumstances,"[1] guidelines have been developed to reduce unwanted variation in medical care, set standards for practice, and improve clinical outcomes. Many studies have reported that CPGs, if followed, can improve clinical standards and the quality of health care.[1-9]

Though more user-friendly and easier to follow than full-text clinical practice guidelines, paper-and-pencil algorithms still must overcome problems with compliance and implementation.[10] These two factors have led to less than favorable reports concerning the usefulness of CPGs.[3] In most cases when guidelines are adequately implemented, as shown in a meta-analyses by Grimshaw and Russell,[3] clinical outcomes improve. Conversely, if guidelines are underutilized or not used at all, or if compliance dwindles over time, they cannot reach their full potential for improving patient care.[4,24-28]

Most obstacles to systematic implementation and use of guidelines involve inherent limitations that prevent their immediate availability, practical applicability, and ease of use.[4,24-28] A 1999 review by Cabana et al[29] identifies lack of awareness (in 46 of 76 studies) and familiarity (in 31 studies) as the most commonly reported barriers of physician adherence to guidelines. This finding is consistent with a major weakness of clinical practice guidelines, which is that they are often in the format of a lengthy document that must be read and adhered to by a physician. They are, therefore, not user-friendly, or are difficult to follow. The fact that CPGs require significant time and effort to reference and follow greatly hinders their implementation and compliance. Factors most likely to increase guidelines' usefulness and achieve improved physician compliance are allowing for immediate access and ease of use during patient care. Toward this end, the format of CPGs must be modified and adapted to meet structural and systemic encumbrances.[30]

Clinical Algorithms

More recently, algorithms or decision trees have been developed to assist in clinical decision making. Operating like a flow chart, algorithms are guides to stepwise evaluation and management strategies that define specific observations to be made, the observations on which subsequent decisions should be based, and finally the recommended steps to be taken.[10] Clinical algorithms are more specific than guide-lines and have been shown to bring about faster learning and improved compliance than guidelines that are in lengthy text form.[10] Many studies have shown that al-gorithms are beneficial in medical settings and can improve clinical practice.[11–23]

It is generally recognized that the development of algorithms has significant promise as an intervention for improving clinical practice patterns in the man-agement of a number of medical conditions. Although algorithms offer im-provements over guidelines and have become increasingly available for common medical conditions, they are not sufficiently used in nonresearch settings, and their promise as an effective intervention to optimize clinical practice and reduce unnecessary variation has yet to come to fruition. One particular problem that is currently being addressed is the utility-limiting static nature of "paper-and-pencil" algorithms.[30] The difficulties encountered with such design are pro-nounced in the current, constantly changing medical-research environment. Up-dating pencil-and-paper algorithms to meet new standards and incorporate new findings is a significant issue, as are practical methods of dissemination. Addi-tionally, it is difficult to assess compliance with the algorithms and their impact on patient care. Researchers must address these implementation issues if they hope to reap the benefits that widespread use of algorithms would generate.

As developers attempt to address the aforementioned difficulties in their de-sign and implementation, the use of algorithmic formats when designing meth-ods of physician practice transformation continues to grow. Computerized decision support systems have the potential to overcome many of the algorithmic imple-mentation issues that have plagued researchers to date. Clear evidence from recent studies has shown that physician use of and compliance with guidelines and algo-rithms is improved when they are presented in a computerized format.[8,31,32]

Computerized Decision Support Systems

Computer use has already permeated many aspects of the business side of med-ical practice. The potential of computers to assist in clinical care entails their in-tegration into areas involving patient care as well. Thus, the potential for the computerization of decision support tools to overcome the problems that have limited the use of paper-and-pencil clinical tools is apparent.[32] In departing from the static-bound constraints of hard-copy text algorithms, a computerized format can be a dynamic, interactive, user-friendly clinical decision support system used at the time of patient care. CDSSs are the next step in this direction.

Computers have the vast potential to provide an extensive and varied network of support to physicians in many areas of clinical practice. By utilizing a com-puterized clinical management/decision support system, immense amounts of in-formation can be instantaneously available to the physician. Such computerized formats can integrate patient-specific information, such as drug allergies, symp-tom severity, functional ability, previous and current medication regime, age, weight, and lab results with evidence-based medical information in determining the most appropriate treatment. Documentation can also be automated and can record a patient's condition and course of care over time. Computerized medication algorithms are capable of tracking a patient's progress and providing information regarding a patient's medications and condition, readily available at the moment of intervention, regardless of provider. In this way, a computerized algorithm promotes continuity of care even when a patient sees a new physician. Specific treatment sequences and tactical recommendations (i.e., dosing ranges and length of pharmacological interventions based on the patient's phase of treatment, and recommended therapeutic blood levels for individual medications) advise the physician in the clinical management of a specific patient. Medication options for the primary syndrome, and strategies for augmenting or changing medications and/or dose can be conveniently displayed in a computer-based algorithm. In addition, information on critical decision points in time for modifying the dose and sub-routines for the treatment of associated symptoms and side effects can also be made available.

Though some researchers recognized the revolutionary potential of computers in clinical settings as early as the 1970s, most of the research into CDSSs has been done within the last 10 years. Multiple studies of computerized guidelines and algorithms have illustrated not only improved physician adherence, but also improved clinical performance and patient outcome as well.[8,13,31–46] To date, the form and nature of computer interventions have been varied. Studies have examined CDSSs and found positive results in a variety of medical venues, e.g., emergency room treatment,[13] intensive care units,[13] tertiary care hospitals,[38] and ambulatory care.[40] Strong evidence reveals exceptional promise in the areas of pharmacology,[36–45] follow-up, and preventive care.[31,47–51] In a meta-analysis of studies using computer support for determining drug dose, Walton et al[43] found a reduction in the time needed to reach therapeutic control, even when total drug use was unchanged, and a lower incidence of negative side effects. The authors suggested that computer support may give physicians the confidence to use higher doses when needed, and help them adjust the drug dose more accurately. Pestotnik et al[36] and Evans et al[37] found that CDSSs improved antibiotic use and clinical outcomes, significantly decreasing adverse drug events and mortality rates. Two studies by Bates et al[38,42] found that the use of physician computer order entry statistically decreased medication errors by significant amounts.

In a comprehensive meta-analysis by Hunt et al,[39] information was compiled for 68 controlled trials using CDSSs. In their review, the authors reported their findings for subgroups of studies, classifying each CDSS as a dosing system, a diagnostic aid, a preventive care system, or other medical care. They found a significant improvement in physician performance in 66% (43/65) of the studies. The authors found that CDSSs enhanced clinical performance for drug dosing, preventive care, and other medical care, though not in diagnosis. The evidence of benefit prompted the authors to make several recommendations for clinical practices. They unequivocally suggested that if possible, such practices implement preventive care reminder systems. They cautioned that dosing CDSSs only be used in systems that would allow for close monitoring. They recommended that, at a minimum, physician adherence rates be assessed, and stressed the importance of in-house evaluation of any new system. The authors also noted that assessment of patient outcome was markedly absent and is an area that warrants further study. They acknowledge that cost could be a prohibitive factor for earlier research, but expect that newer CDSSs should allow greater ease for such patient outcomes evaluation. In their review, Hunt et al limited the inclusion of CDSS studies examined to those meeting specific design parameters. Only studies of interventions involving the use of CDSSs in a clinical setting, by a healthcare practitioner, and those that also included a control group comparison with the CDSS were included. These stipulations for inclusion in their review are especially relevant to our approach since they mirror the parameters of our system. The conclusion drawn by Hunt et al regarding the usefulness and the potential for specific CDSSs is one measuring stick by which we have evaluated our ability to overcome the limitations of previous designs and maximize the factors most indicative of a positive outcome.

In the area of behavioral health care, where pharmacology and preventive care play a very important role, we are beginning to realize the potential of CDSSs.

Computerized Decision Support Systems in Clinical Psychiatry

Unfortunately, a majority of studies report that patients treated for major psychiatric disorders routinely receive suboptimal care.[52–59] Thus, there is a conspicuous need for improved standards of care in behavioral health care. In identifying the key areas of deficiency, it is evident that there exists significant potential for improving patient outcomes if an effective method of influencing physicians practice patterns can be identified. In the field of behavioral health care, as in others, accurate treatment and drug selection can shorten the duration of acute care treatment. Additionally, efficacy studies indicate that patients who receive optimal care in the acute phase of treatment have the best long-term prognosis.[52,53]

These deficiencies are prominent in various stages of treatment. For example, many patients treated for major depressive disorder are not given an adequate dose of medication, or are not treated long enough to optimally benefit from the treatment.[54–57] Similarly, despite recent advances in newer, safer psychotropic medications that have fewer side effects and fewer long-term effects, these drugs are often not used adequately, if at all.[52,54,58,60] In other cases, patients who receive medications that require blood levels and other monitoring often do not receive appropriate follow-up care.[59]

As mentioned earlier, CDSSs have shown exceptional promise in the areas of pharmacology and preventive care. CDSSs can make new pharmaceutical research findings significantly more accessible, and allow information and recommendations about medication treatments to be readily available at the time of treatment. This can encourage the use of new medications that have fewer side effects and long-term effects as well as provide information concerning proper usage, such as how to prescribe the medication, and proper follow-up care. The computerized recommendations and reminders can advise the physician and provide valuable support to the caregiver.

We are beginning to realize the potential of computer medication algorithms/CDSSs for improving medication choice and dose, reducing medication error, improving preventive and follow-up care, and, in general, improving the overall quality and efficiency of clinical practice. For these tools to aid physicians, it is essential that they be well designed and have pragmatic application, keeping in mind physicians' needs and methods of everyday practice.

Considerations Important in the Software Design

To be implemented, computer medication algorithms/CDSSs must be practical and be appealing to practitioners. As such, they must be extremely user-friendly and not distracting, such that they provide a framework for thinking about clinical problems without adding to the work load. They must support clinical work flow, and not restrict the practice or physician autonomy. Computer displays should be simple, direct, and easy to use, with direct access to patient information, progress notes, and order of computer flow and entry of patient information. If designed well, by keeping practitioners needs at the forefront, these tools will have the potential to not only improve practice patterns and clinical outcomes, but also reduce physician work load and paperwork. Patient information security is another concern of physicians and patients that must be addressed by a CDSS. Physicians understand the importance of patient confidentiality, and they expect to maintain privacy of their records. It is essential that CDSSs protect records from unauthorized disclosure, and that they are capable of selectively allowing varying levels of access for different users based on user-defined security levels. To meet the challenge of ensuring confidentiality, CDSSs must incorporate security measures that will protect records, and these measures will have to be upgraded periodically to meet legal requirements and technical advances.

Computer systems are widely used in medicine today. A CDSS should be able to integrate and interface with current electronic infrastructure and available databases. It must be capable of importing and exporting data and files; it must allow for interfacing with other computerized systems and, if necessary, it must have the ability to launch other applications. In addition, since it is essential for CDSSs to be designed as tools to be used at the point of care, a portable computer module may be required. CDSSs will have to be capable of network connection to a database server, either by a data port or modem.

The Computerized Treatment Algorithm

At the University of Texas Southwestern Medical Center at Dallas, we are currently developing a computerized decision-support software (the computerized treatment algorithm, CTA). The literature reviewed thus far has been extremely instructive and insightful for many aspects of the design during the development process. In thinking about the functional logistics of implementation as well as the specifications of the actual software and user interface, we have developed a platform that fulfills essential parameters defined by the research to date, and which improves upon previous CDSSs. The current CDSS is designed to incorporate the key elements we have highlighted in this chapter, as well as those identified in the literature.

The CTA application is a clinical support tool designed to assist in the treatment and management of clinical care for patients with psychiatric disorders. The current, fully functional version of our software program can be loaded onto any personal computer meeting the recommended system requirements. The program applies the logical principles underlying the clinical algorithms used in the Texas Medication Algorithm Project (TMAP)[61] to individualized patient data to assist a physician in providing optimal treatment for each patient.

Development

The CTA program was developed in collaboration with software developers from UT Southwestern (UTSW) Medical Center Clinical Information Services (CIS). Internally, the CTA application consists of three separate tiers responsible for user interaction, decision-tree reasoning, and the storage of clinical data. The functional relationships between the three tiers (or parts) of the CTA program can be described as follows:

The user interface: This user interface is an interactive application written for the Microsoft Windows platform and is developed using Visual Basic programming language. The user can navigate through Web-like buttons, which provide a user-friendly environment in which to work. It utilizes ActiveX and OCX technology, and graphical display of data elements is provided through the charting interface licensed from Quinn-Curtis. The user interface is the only application of the CTA program that is visible to the user.

The rules engine: The clinical algorithms used by TMAP have been translated into specific rules, compiled into a knowledge base, and then implemented using the industry-standard logical inference engine licensed from Blaze Software. The rules engine application operates behind the user interface to apply the TMAP algorithms to the current and historical patient data. It provides treatment options to the physician via the user interface.

The database: All clinical information entered into the CTA application is stored securely in the back-end SQL server. The database also stores user-specific data (for limiting access to clinical information), as well as the reference tables for medications and doses. Because both the reference tables and the rules knowledge base by which the rules engine processes the patient information is stored on a central server, updates to the algorithms can be implemented through the server, without user intervention.

System Requirements

CTA was designed as a client/server application, capable of supporting multiple local/remote clients. However, the CTA application can also be deployed in a single-user environment where a single PC can run all of the client and server components. Listed below are the minimum recommended configurations and software requirements for the machines:

Client personal computer (PC):
Hardware: IBM compatible, Pentium 100 processor, 32-megabyte (MB) random access memory (RAM), and 50 MB free hard disk space.
Software: Windows 9x/NT/2000 with Microsoft Explorer 5.0 TCP/IP connectivity to the server.

Server computer:
Hardware: IBM compatible, Pentium 400 processor, minimum 128-MB RAM, minimum 2 gigabytes of hard disk space.
Software: Windows NT Server 4.0/2000, SQL Server 7.x

Conclusion

We believe that a computerized treatment algorithm is a viable solution to the obstacles confronting physicians today, and is a logical progression in the methodology toward use of new technological advancements in behavioral health care. We are developing a computerized treatment algorithm that promises to reduce error, improve clinical outcomes, improve standards of practice, incorporate new medical therapies into practice, reduce unwanted variation in practice, and ultimately make clinical practice more effective. Further development that incorporates multiple treatment algorithms for both psychiatric and medical illnesses can easily be accomplished. Several plug-in efforts with other informatics systems are also under way.

References

1. Committee to Advise the Public Health Service on Clinical Practice Guidelines, Institute of Medicine, Field MJ, Lohr KN, eds. *Clinical Practice Guidelines: Directions of a New Program.* Washington, DC: National Academy Press, 1990.
2. Katon W, Von Korff M, Lin E, et al. Collaborative management to achieve treatment guidelines: impact on depression in primary care. *JAMA* 1995;273:1026–1031.
3. Grimshaw JM, Russell IA. Effect of clinical guidelines on medical practice: a systematic review of rigorous evaluations. *Lancet* 1993;342:1317–1322.
4. Lomas JL, Anderson JM, Dominick-Pierre K, Vayda E, Enkin MW, Hannah WJ. Do practice guidelines guide practice? The effect of a consensus statement on the practice of physicians. *N Engl J Med* 1989;321:1307–1311.
5. Lubarsky DA, Glass PS, Ginsberg B, et al. The successful implementation of pharmaceutical practice guidelines: analysis of associated outcomes and cost savings. *Anesthesiology* 1997;86:1145–1160.
6. Nestor A, Calhoun AC, Dickson M, Kalick C. Cross-sectional analysis of the relationship between national guideline recommended asthma drug therapy and emergency/hospital use within a managed care population. *Ann Allergy Asthma Immunol* 1998;81:327–330.

7. Webb LZ, Kuykendall DH, Zeiger RS, et al. The impact of status asthmaticus practice guidelines on patient outcome and physician behavior. *QRB* 1992;471–476.
8. Lobach DF, Hammond WE. Computerized decision support based on a clinical practice guidelines improves compliance with care standards. *Excerpta Med* 1997;102: 89–98.
9. Lohr KN, Brook RH. Quality of care in episodes of respiratory illness among Medicaid patients in New Mexico. *Acad Clin* 1980;92:99–106.
10. Hadorn DC, McCormick K, Diokno A. An annotated algorithm approach to clinical guideline development. *JAMA* 1992;267:3311–3314.
11. Schoenbaum SC, Gottlieb LK. Algorithm based improvement of clinical quality. *Br Med J* 1990;301:1374–1377.
12. Trivedi MH, Bebattista C, Fawcett J, et al. Developing treatment algorithms for unipolar depression in cyberspace: International Psychopharmacology Project (IPAP). *Psychopharmacol Bull* 1998;34:355–359.
13. Goldman L, Weinberg M. A computer-derived protocol to aid in the diagnosis of emergency room patients with acute chest pain. *N Engl J Med* 1982;307:588–593.
14. Nerlich M, Maghsudi M. Algorithms for early management of pelvic fractures. *Injury* 1996;27:29–37.
15. Rossi-Mori A, Pisanelli DM, Ricci FL. Evaluation stages and design steps for knowledge-based systems in medicine. *Med Inf* 1990;15:191–204.
16. Kassirer JP, Borry GA. Clinical problem solving: a behavioral analysis. In: Reggia JA, Tuhrim S, eds. *Computer-assisted Medical Decision Making,* vol 2. New York: Springer-Verlag, 1985:85–107.
17. Bridgeman T, Flores M, Rosenbluth J, Pierog J. One emergency department's experience: clinical algorithms and documentation. *J Emerg Nurs* 1997;23:316–325.
18. Bogaerts J, Vuylsteke B, Martinez-Tello W, et al. Simple algorithms for the management of genital ulcers: evaluation in a primary health care centre in Kigali, Rwanda. *Bull WHO* 1995;73:761–767.
19. Ashraf H, Bhan MK, Bhatnagar S, et al. Evaluation of an algorithm for the treatment of persistent diarrhea: a multicentre study. *Bull WHO* 1996;74:479–489.
20. Christy C, McConnochie KM, Zernik N, Brzoza S. Impact of an algorithm-guided nurse intervention on the use of immunization opportunities. *Arch Pediatr Adolesc Med* 1997;151:384–391.
21. Hunt Johnson M, Moroney CE, Gay CF. Relieving nausea and vomiting in patients with cancer: a treatment algorithm. *Oncol Nurs Forum* 1997;24:53–57.
22. McKinley BA, Parmley CL, Tonneson AS. Standardized management of intracranial pressure: a preliminary clinical trial. *J Trauma Injury Infect Crit Care.* 1999;46:271–279.
23. Gilbert K. An algorithm for diagnosis and treatment of status epilepticus in adults. *J Neurosci Nurs* 1999;31:34–36.
24. Davis DA, Taylor-Vaisey A. Translating guidelines into practice: a systematic review of theoretic concepts, practical experience and research in the adoption of clinical practice guidelines. *Can Med Assoc J* 1997;157:408–416.
25. Greco PJ, Eisenberg JM. Changing physicians' practices. *N Engl J Med* 1993;320: 1271–1274.
26. Pathman DE, Konrad TR, Freed GL, Freeman VA, Koch GG. The awareness-to-adherence model of the steps to clinical guideline compliance: the case of pediatric vaccine recommendations. *Med Care* 1996;34:873–889.
27. Flocke SA, Stange KC, Fedirko TL. Dissemination of information about the US Preventive Service Task Force guidelines. *Arch Fam Med* 1994;3:1006–1008.

28. Gupta L, Ward JE, Hayward R. Clinical practice guidelines in clinical practice: a national survey of recall, attitudes and impact. *Med J Aust* 1997;166:69–72.
29. Cabana MD, Rand CS, Powe NR, et al. Why don't physicians follow clinical practice guidelines? A framework for improvement. *JAMA* 1999;282(15):1458–1465.
30. Abendroth TW, Greenes RA. Computer presentation of clinical algorithms. *MD Comput* 1989;6:295–299.
31. Johnston ME, Langston KB, Haynes RB, Mathieu A. Effects of computer-based decision support systems on clinician performance and patient outcome. *Ann Intern Med* 1994;120:135–142.
32. Elson RB, Connelly DP. Computerized patient records in primary care: their role in mediating guideline-driven physician behavior change. *Arch Fam Med* 1995;4:698–705.
33. Sullivan F, Mitchell E. Has practitioner computing made a difference to patient care? A systematic review of published reports. *Br Med J* 1995;311:848–852.
34. Litzelman DK, Dittas RS, Miller ME, Tierney WM. Requiring physicians to respond to computerized reminders improves their compliance with preventative care protocols. *J Intern Med* 1993;8:311–317.
35. Chambers CV, Valban DJ, Lepidus Cralson B, Ungemack JA, Grasberger DM. Microcomputer-generated reminders: improving the compliance of primary care physicians with mammography screening guidelines. *J Fam Pract* 1989;29:273–280.
36. Pestotnik SL, Classen DC, Evans RS, Burke JP. Implementing antibiotic practice guidelines through computer-assisted decision support: clinical and financial outcomes. *Ann Intern Med* 1996;124:884–890.
37. Evans RS, Pestotnik SL, Classen DC, et al. A computer-assisted management program for antibiotics and other antiinfective agents. *N Engl J Med* 1998;338:232–238.
38. Bates DW, Leape LL, Cullen DJ, et al. Effect of computerized physician order entry on prevention of serious medication errors. *JAMA* 1998;280:1311–1316.
39. Hunt DL, Haynes BH, Hanna SE, Smith K. Effects of computer-based clinical decision support systems of physician performance and patient outcomes. *JAMA* 1998;280:1339–1346.
40. Cannon SR, Gardner RM. Experience with a computerized interactive protocol system using HELP. *Comput Biomed Res* 1980;13:399–409.
41. Chantellier G, Columbet I, Degoulet P. Computer-adjusted dosage of anticoagulant therapy improves the quality of anticoagulation. *Med Inf* 1998;9:819–823.
42. Bates DW, Teich JM, Lee J, et al. The impact of computerized physician order entry on medication error prevention. *J Am Med Inf Assoc* 1999;6:313–321.
43. Walton R, Dovey S, Harvey E, Freemantle N. Computer support for determining drug dose: systematic review and meta-analysis. *Br Med J* 1999;318:984–990.
44. Poller L, Shiach CR, MacCallum PK, et al. Multicentre randomised study of computerised anticoagulant dosage. European Concerted Action on Anticoagulation. *Lancet* 1998;352:1505–1509.
45. Fitzmaurice DA, Hobbs FD, Murray ET. Primary care anticoagulant clinic management using computerized decision support and near patient International Normalized Ratio (INR) testing: routine data from a practice nurse-led clinic. *Fam Pract* 1998;15:144–146.
46. McDonald CJ. Use of a computer to detect and respond to clinical events: its effect on clinician behavior. *Ann Intern Med* 1976;84:162–167.
47. Frame PS, Zimmer JG, Werth PL, Hall WJ, Eberly SW. Computer-based verses manual health maintenance tracking: a controlled trial. *Arch Fam Med* 1994;3:581–588.

48. Ornstein SM, Garr DR, Jenkins RG, Rust PF, Arnon A. Computer-generated physician and patient reminders: tools to improve population adherence to selected preventative services. *J Fam Pract* 1991;32:82–90.
49. McPhee SJ, Bird JA, Fordham D, Rodnick JE, Osborn EH. Promoting cancer prevention activities by primary care physicians: results of a randomized, controlled trial. *JAMA* 1991;266:538–544.
50. Turner BJ. A controlled trial of strategies to improve delivery of preventative care. *Proc Annu Conf Res Med Educ* 1987;26:9–13.
51. Harris RP, O'Malley MS, Fletcher SW, Knight BP. Prompting physicians for preventative procedures: a five-year study of manual and computer reminders. *Am J Prev Med* 1990;6:145–152.
52. Public Health Service Agency for Health Care Policy and Research. *Depression in Primary Care: Treatment of Major Depression.* AHCPR publication 93-051. Rockville, MD: US Dept of Health and Human Resources, 1993:2.
53. Rush AJ, Trivedi MH. Treating depression to remission. *Psychiatr Ann* 1995;25:704–709.
54. Hirschfield RM, Keller MB, Panico S, et al. The national depressive and manic-depressive association consensus statement on the undertreatment of depression. *JAMA* 1997;277:333–340.
55. Parikh SV, Lesage AD, Kennedy SH, Goering ON. Depression in Ontario: undertreatment and factors relayed to depression use. *J Affect Disord* 1999;52:67–76.
56. Eisenberg L. Treating depression and anxiety in primary care: closing the gap between knowledge and practice. *N Engl J Med* 1992;326:1080–1084.
57. Friedman RA, Kocsis JH. Pharmacotherapy for chronic depression. *Psychiatr Clin North Am* 1996;19:121–132.
58. Casey D. The relationship of pharmacology to side effects. *J Clin Psychiatry* 1997;58:55–62.
59. Marcus SC, Olfson M, Pincus HA, Zarin DA, Kupfer DJ. Therapeutic drug monitoring of mood stabilizers in Medicaid patients with bipolar disorder. *Am J Psychiatry* 1999;156:1014–1018.
60. Galvin PM, Knezek LD, Rush AJ, Toprac MG, Johnson B. Clinical and economic impact of newer verses older antipsychotic medications in a community health center. *Clin Ther* 1999;21:1105–1116.
61. Crimson LM, Trivedi MH, Pigott TA, et al. The Texas Medication Algorithm Project: Report of the Texas Consensus Conference Panel on the medication treatment of major depressive disorder. *J Clin Psychiatry* 1999;60:142–156.

Part III
Consumers' Issues

Introduction

RICHARD THOMPSON AND ELLEN GRAVES

We are in the midst of an information and technology revolution called the Internet. According to *Cyber Dialogue*, "By 2005, 88.5 million adults will use the Internet to find health information, shop for health products, and communicate with affiliated payors and providers through online channels. The consumer demand for healthcare content has already reached critical mass—an estimated 36.7 million adults—and will continue to grow at roughly twice the rate of the overall online population."

The Internet can become an ally for providers, a tool that physicians can use to better meet their patients' needs for consumer health information and therefore, increase patient satisfaction and compliance. According to *Cyber Dialogue*'s "Cybercitizen Health 2000," 61% of consumers want their physician to recommend a Web site for health information, but only 4% actually learn about Web sites from their provider.

A solution in the near term may require office-based physicians, clinics, and hospitals to merge computer-based patient education solutions with those that are Web-based. The computer-based solution can allow the provider to edit the patient education content to include Internet URLs in notes at the end of a handout. This health information becomes a "patient education Rx." The URLs would be disease or procedure-specific information that would augment the handout and guide patients to either the provider's own Web site or Web sites he or she recommends.

Our vision of the future includes Internet healthcare portals that can be accessed with an information prescription from a patient's physician. The patient will log on to the site, answer questions such as gender, age, disease, medications, and language, and then be guided to relevant patient education information. This information will be linked to a variety of formats, including snippets of video, animation, and audio, as well as clinical information, such as abstracts and current articles. Other links will include access to consumer advocates, medical providers designated as patient coaches, and on-line communities of peers who have similar health problems. Such portals will be peer reviewed and meet patient privacy requirements.

The chapters in this section focus on the forces that have propelled patients to become consumers of health care, and the issues involved in helping older adults use computers to access the growing availability of behavioral health information technologies.

6

Behavioral Health Consumerism and the Internet

NORMAN ALESSI AND MILTON HUANG

One of the most significant consequences of Internet development has been in the area of consumer health care. Recent research found evidence of upward of 25 million adults in the United States searching for health information and potentially 15,000 health care sites.[1] Never in the history of medicine have patients had such ready access to medical knowledge or such an ability to communicate with a broad range of similarly or identically ill patients, regardless of disease rarity.[2] This is a new era in the development of medicine and mental health care. Nevertheless, there are potential downsides to this evolution. Issues of security and confidentiality are the concerns most frequently cited, but they are also the most obvious. This chapter discusses Web development in relationship to computer–human interfaces as well as managed care, the forces that have propelled patients into increasingly becoming healthcare consumers, the periods of Web development based on the prevailing technologies of the time and the associated functions, as they became available to consumers, and future trends in Internet development.

The Internet/The Web

The Internet, in its current "Web browser" format, is a significant information technology because of its adaptation speed and economic impact, and the resulting development of industries. The development of the Web browser provided a significant computer–human interface that facilitates access to an overwhelming volume of information, including health-related information for consumers and healthcare professionals.

Prior to the Web browser's introduction, the Internet had existed for a number of decades as a popular, yet not publicly available, advanced communication protocol. The TCP/IP (Transmission Control Protocol/Internet Protocol) was developed in large part as a military response to potential warfare and due to a need for continuous distribution of information, regardless of communication interruptions. Thus the packet-based distribution methodology was born with its associated IP addressing.

Prior to the development of the modern Web, desktop computers used the popular and user-friendly Graphics User Interface (GUI), which allowed a greater number of people access to computers. Before its advent, nearly all computer users had to have prior training or a compelling interest in computer science, as using the software and hardware required expertise. These limitations led to only a relative few who invested the time and money in pre-GUI desktop units. Although the GUI was a marked improvement by allowing greater access, the cost of software packages, applications, and informational sources was still prohibitive. From a consumer standpoint, the number of software packages concerning mental health was limited, and were often bundled into general medical software packages. These were often used for short periods before the user became uninterested in the content and had to either buy newer versions or abandon the software altogether. Although far from perfect, it was a reasonable introduction of computers to the consumer population.

The Web and Managed Care

The Web, as we refer to the Internet, has had a profound effect on mental health and medicine in general that is well worth noting. Medicine has undergone profound changes in the last decade. Managed care has been the most influential force and has affected the delivery of care and altered the roles and the relationship of the patient and physician. Psychiatry and mental health have been affected much more than other areas of medicine, because twice the number of people are enrolled in behavioral managed care programs than in medical HMOs. Several limitations have been introduced, including shortened stays on inpatient units, the unavailability of long-term institutionalization for the most impaired, and decreased numbers of sessions in outpatient clinics. The use of paraprofessionals as physician extenders to decrease cost, selecting medications for the treatment of disorders based on cost containment, clinical care guidelines, and the decreased use of psychotherapy are just a few of the alterations that have occurred in response to the need for cost containment. Some, but not all, of these changes have been positive. In fact, a major consequence has been to make patients turn to self-help, though not necessarily by choice, and not always in their best interests. The Web has empowered patients when they felt the most abandoned.

The Web is a fusion of networking and the desktop computer that serves as an extension of the GUI, which has extended computer availability to so many. With the networking provided via the TCP/IP protocol, we now have an unlimited wealth of knowledge that had been obtainable only by those with big budgets.

From Patients to Consumers

The need for self-help has become more prevalent over the last 10 to 15 years in all medical areas, especially in mental health. Driven by a sense of abandonment, patients have become more likely to seek self-help information, thus attracting the interest of information providers. This self-help movement has been supported by the print media (books and magazines), video- and audiotapes, and infomercials. These media have made healthcare information widely available. Unfortunately, in addition to being wooed by conscientious members of the medical information industry, the patient, as consumer, has now become potential prey for unscrupulous sellers who want to capture them for fiduciary gain. Because of all the medical information available on the Web to patients, both good and bad, the Web has the potential to be both a positive and a negative force, in that patients have become both consumers and victims.

The patient's and the consumer's domains are markedly different. Consumers are not protected by the status of "patient" and the Hippocratic oath, but rather are subject to those who would conspire to sell them anything, and they must now live by the customer oath of "buyer beware."

In addition to the managed care environment, other factors that have fostered the increase in healthcare information on the Internet include the aging of the population, the increase in the population's education levels, and the demand for higher quality care and goods.[3–6] Internet-savvy consumers now demand results quickly. Today's world operates in time defined not by the clocks of our parents' generation, but by those of the Internet generation.

The Evolution of the Web and Mental Health

The Web is a highly volatile growth area that has impact on technology, psychology, sociology, philosophy, and economics, among other fields. At the core of the Web's evolution are several identifiable periods during which technologies and applications have defined the resulting functionality. The identified periods are (1) home pages and sites, (2) portals, and (3) e-commerce. During each period specific resources became available to consumers. As we discuss these periods we will mention the business models that the Web has either influenced or been the source of.

Period 1—Home Pages and Sites

This period introduced the browser as the interface for the Internet. Home pages in mental health often originated from professional organizations, such as the American Academy of Child and Adolescent Psychiatry (AACAP) (www.aacap. org), the American Psychological Association (www.apa.org), and American Psychiatric Association (www.psych.org). Academic departments of psychiatry, psychology, social work, and counseling, such as the University of Michigan (www.psych.med.umcih.edu), Harvard University (http://www.hmcnet.harvard. edu/psych/index.html), and Auckland in Australia (http://www.auckland.ac.nz/ pbsc/mpshome.html), had sites often starting at a mere one to two pages. Individuals also created their own sites, such as Dr. Bob's (http://uhs.bsd.uchicago. edu/~bhsiung/mental.html) and Milton Huang (http://www.psych.med.umich. edu/web/UMpsych/staff/mhuang/papers.htm). There were few development tools or Web site conceptualization models. Almost all work was done by hand coding. Tens of thousands of visits to a site was thought to be a significant number; few realized the potential growth of the Web.

This period rapidly evolved from Web pages to Web sites. These sites could become extremely large, often encompassing hundreds of pages, thus becoming unwieldy and difficult to navigate. Search tools soon made navigating easier, allowing for word-by-word searches through sites or the entire Internet. After these developments came an increased use of e-mail and chat rooms, means by which consumers could communicate with others.

During this period consumers had the following:

- Access to information: A few sites provided access to psychiatric diagnoses and treatment descriptions. Consumers could do Medline literature searches using PubMed (http://www.ncbi.nlm.nih.gov/PubMed/overview.html). Consumers had the ability to access information that had previously been available only to professionals.
- The ability to diagnose one's own illnesses. Sites offered checklists that enabled consumers to diagnose a potential illness. Many sites gave in-depth comparisons between different illnesses, allowing patients to grasp the strengths and weaknesses of the diagnostic process.
- Sites that offered consumer-based information, in several languages, such as AACAP's "Facts for Families." The Web, even at this stage of development, demonstrated its potential to make all knowledge global, a trend that continues today in all sectors. The Web was increasingly becoming the standard for worldwide communication.

Period 2—Portals and Sharing

Due to the magnitude of information that was becoming available, sites that specialized in bringing together multiple sites were developed to serve as a Web user's "home base." The first site to effectively use portal technology was Yahoo. This site enabled users to search many sites, thereby making it easier to access specific information. A number of vertical portals have developed over the years that specialize in medical and mental health. The vertical ports initially only brought sites together, but over time became the mechanism by which medical news was distributed.

The utilization of databases became increasingly common. They enabled users to systematically search through and collect large volumes of information.

Another significant implementation has been that of communication-based technologies, such as e-mail, chat rooms, Internet-based telephony, and video conferencing. These technologies once required monthly service fees but are now often free with the purchase of a computer.

This period was characterized by the following:

- Increasing access to state-of-the-art medical information from a vast number of sources[7–11]: Portals such as Medscape, WebMD, and DrKoop.com made medical information increasingly easy to access.[12] Furthermore, patients could customize their entry into a portal by implementing databases and data warehousing, thus accessing medical information that is relevant to their condition.

- The availability of hospitals, healthcare systems, and doctors' profiles Web sites[13]: Consumers could now investigate any healthcare provider, which helped in choosing a practitioner.
- Consumers could share their experiences, concerns, and fears with others with similar illnesses. This function filled the void left because of managed care's impact on the doctor–patient relationship.
- Patients could seek additional assistance through facilitated communication via telephony, email, and Internet-based teleconferencing.
- Electronic patient records could now be used more frequently by healthcare delivery systems. Issues of security, confidentiality, and privacy became more important.

Period 3—E-Commerce

The Internet evolved from a medium of information exchange into a new form of commerce. Not only were sites being used for the purpose of advertising, as evidenced by the pervasive use of banners, they became a form of business that rivaled traditional forms of commerce. Numerous companies have developed in an attempt to take advantage of the most significant evolutions in business modeling to occur during the 20th century.

This period was characterized by the following:

- The availability of prescription medications on-line[14]: Consumers could now provide information to physicians who assess, diagnose, and in some cases prescribe medications and treatments on-line.
- Medical portals could provide consumers with customized healthcare and disease-related information. In addition, advertising banners are displayed to consumers offering the opportunity to purchase medically related texts, newsletters, videos, and audio materials.
- Medical portals could provide click-through opportunities for consumers to purchase healthy "natural" herbal medical preparations. Leading pharmacies also provide banners and associated discounts for medications purchased on-line.

Consumer Health Care Areas of the Future and the Internet

The Internet will continue to provide consumer healthcare.[15,16] A number of areas will continue to be significant.

Quality of Information

As more information concerning health care and personal well-being becomes available to consumers, its quality becomes increasingly important.[17,18] Who will define and distribute quality information consumers?[19,20] What will be the role of medical professional organizations such as the American Psychiatric Association, and AACAP? Will there be a role for national or federal regulation of the information available to healthcare consumers?[21]

Doctor–Patient Relationship

An important component of care will always be the effective communication between a patient and the caregiver. Given the intrusions of managed care and other major cultural trends, the ability of clinicians to engage the patient's trust has become quite challenging.[22] The Internet may serve both clinicians and patients well by developing and maintaining that trust. How will the use of the Internet by consumers influence their ability to trust their care providers? What role can clinicians play in helping to develop trust in an Internet-based healthcare delivery system?[23]

Identification and Access of Relevant Information

As information sources abound, the identification and access to relevant medical information will become increasingly important. How good are our current search engines?[24] How will patients' mental health conditions, such as depression, Alzheimer's, and anxiety or thought disorders, influence their access to information?

The Role of Patient as Consumer vs. Healthcare Consumer

No one can question the benefits patients receive by having access to information about their illnesses. Nevertheless, a healthcare consumer will be treated differently from a patient. What will be the strategies of managed care corporations, Web portals, healthcare delivery systems, and other for-profit institutions in attempting to recruit patients?[25,26] How will consumers determine if there is added value? Employers, providers, payers, and managed care organizations will have to rethink how they work in an Internet-based medical economic environment.

Internet-Based Care

The Web will allow for increasingly sophisticated interactions. Although it is primarily text based now, it will soon expand to include telephony and video. Will this become the new medium for psychotherapy,[27,28] and will the majority of our work be performed over the Web? These questions demand a reanalysis of our views concerning what constitutes psychopathology and "object relations."[29] New disorders will undoubtedly arise because of this medium, such as "Internet addictions."[30]

Point of Care

Telemedicine, or in this case telepsychiatry/tele–mental health, is described as a means to allow deliver health care at a distance. This formerly involved the use tele-conferencing equipment utilizing ISDN or T1 lines. Plain old telephone service (POTS) has always proven inadequate and allowed the transmission of only single images. Now, with the development of the Internet, video, and technology utilizing multimedia capabilities, this will all change. Where will patients most likely be seen? Undoubtedly, home care and home visits will reemerge.[31–34] This then leads to the following questions: What would be the implications of increasing home-based care, and will this improve the quality of care?[35] State or national boundaries could potentially play a significant role in determining where one receives care.[36]

Electronic Patient Record

A number of fundamental questions are raised by the Internet's potential interactions with medical databases, such as electric patient records. Today, the possibility of having patient records on-line is a reality for many healthcare systems.[37,38] These systems often do not include any mental health data, which is a problem that has not yet reached discussion level. Nevertheless, the basic assumption is that the healthcare system controls the record and its contents.[39] Given that these records will follow patients for life and require information collection from many different sites and healthcare organizations, the fundamental question is: Who should "own" the patients record?[40] This was traditionally determined by the proximity of the patient to a hospital, but this geographical adjacency will not exist much longer. Who will develop the standards for such a "patient-centered" patient record? Services will have to be developed to manage and store these records, and guidelines will have to be introduced to determine who will have access to these records. A government agency will have to oversee the standardization, implementation, and quality of these records. This then leads to the most pressing question: How will confidentiality be maintained for patients if their records are under an agency's control?[41]

The Future of Medicine: The Web

The Web has had a profound impact on consumer healthcare issues. The most important consideration now is how it will impact and influence the future. This is an area of rapid undocumented growth, and certainly neither systematically studied nor researched. Oddly enough, the Internet has grown so rapidly that its history has been largely forgotten. It is a new "prehistoric era" with little to prove its presence, despite its obvious significance.

A number of factors, such as the aging our population, increasing sophistication in the use of information technologies, an increased demand for improved quality of health care, and a desire to be involved in one's healthcare destiny will increase the consumer's demands.[42] Those who can develop the products demanded by the consumer will become leaders in future delivery systems. It is important that we maintain vigilance in this area, for regardless of what consumers may think, care providers will always carry the responsibility for the patient's welfare.

References

1. Bickert M. *The Impact of Ecommerce on Legacy Health-Care Companies.* New York: Cyber Dialogue, 1999.
2. Goldstein D, Flory J. Lasso the power of the Internet. *Infocare* 1997:Jan–Feb:36–40,42.
3. Slack WV. *Cybermedicine.* San Francisco: Jossey-Bass, 1997.
4. Herzlinger R. *Market-Driven Health Care.* Reading, MA: Addison-Wesley, 1997.
5. Hochstein M. Seven societal trends driving consumer interest in the Internet and E-commerce. In: Haylock CF, Muscarella L, eds. *Net Success: 24 Leaders in Web Commerce Show You How to Put the Internet to Work for Your Business.* Holbrook, MA: Adams Media, 1999:16–21.
6. Pringle B. Healthcare: operating in the third dimension. In: Haylock CF, Muscarella L, eds. *Net Success 24 Leaders in Web Commerce Show You How to Put the Internet to Work for Your Business.* Holbrook, MA: Adams Media, 1999:275–286.
7. Gilbert JA. Beyond billboards: building interactive Web sites. *Health Data Manag* 1998;6(12):40–44.
8. Gross V. A women's resource center in a rural setting. *Med Ref Serv Q* 1999; 18(1):25–35.
9. Guard R, Haag D, Kaya B, et al. An electronic consumer health library: NetWellness. *Bull Med Libr Assoc* 1996;84(4):468–477.
10. Lynch C. Medical libraries, bioinformatics, and networked information: a coming convergence? *Bull Med Libr Assoc* 1999;87(4):408–414.
11. Voge S. NOAH—New York Online Access to Health: library collaboration for bilingual consumer health information on the Internet. *Bull Med Libr Assoc* 1998;86(3): 326–334.
12. Menduno M. Net profits. *Hosp Health Netw* 1999;73(3):44–48,50,52.
13. Herreria J. America's Doctor Online provides easy access for consultations. *Profiles Healthcare Mark* 1999;15(1):31–32.
14. Hatfield CL, May SK, Markoff JS. Quality of consumer drug information provided by four Web sites. *Am J Health Syst Pharmacol* 1999;56(22):2308–2311.
15. Cochrane JD. Healthcare @ the speed of thought. *Integr Healthcare Rep* May 1999; 1–14,16–17.
16. Bastian H. The Power of Sharing Knowledge: Consumer Participation in the Cochrane Collaboration. The Cochrane Collaboration. Consumer Advocate, Dec 1994.
17. Lang LA, Shannon TE. Value and choice: providing consumers with information on the quality of health care. Conference overview. *Joint Comm J Qual Improv* 1997; 23(5):231–238.
18. Price SL, Hersh WR. Filtering Web pages for quality indicators: an empirical approach to finding high quality consumer health information on the World Wide Web [In Process Citation]. *Proc AMIA Symp* 1999;(1–2):911–915.
19. Marine S, Guard R, Morris T, et al. A model for enhancing worldwide personal health and wellness. *Medinfo* 1998;9(pt 2):1265–1268.
20. Cronin C. Using the Internet to educate consumers about health care choices. *Manag Care Q* 1998;6(1):29–33.
21. The Advisory Commission on Consumer Protection and Quality in the Health Care

Industry. Improving quality in a changing health care industry. In: *Investing in Information Systems.* Consumer Bill of Rights, Columbia MD. 48 pages. 1998.
22. Mechanic D. Public trust and initiatives for new health care partnerships. *Milbank Q* 1998;76(2):281–302.
23. Bluming A, Mittelman PS. Los Angeles Free-Net: an experiment in interactive telecommunication between lay members of the Los Angeles community and health care experts [see comments]. *Bull Med Libr Assoc* 1996;84(2):217–222.
24. Wu G, Li J. Comparing Web search engine performance in searching consumer health information: evaluation and recommendations. *Bull Med Libr Assoc* 1999;87(4):456–461.
25. Wilkins AS. Expanding Internet access for health care consumers. *Health Care Manag Rev* 1999;24(3):30–41.
26. Warson A. Managing patient demand on-line. *Med Interface* 1997;10(3):80–84.
27. Pergament D. Internet psychotherapy: current status and future regulation. *Health Matrix* 1998;8(2):233–279.
28. Seemann O, unter Mitarbeit N, Michel N. et al. Psybertherapy on the Internet and its implications for psychiatry, psychotherapy, and psychosomatics. *Eur J Med Res* 1998;3(12):571–576.
29. Clarke B. Psychotherapy under construction. Can telepsychiatric and online services mirror the traditional counseling experience? *Behav Healthcare Tomorrow* 1999;8(1): 36,38–40.
30. Stein DJ. Internet addiction, Internet psychotherapy [letter; comment]. *Am J Psychiatry* 1997;154(6):890.
31. Chepesiuk R. Making house calls: using telecommunications to bring health care into the home. *Environ Health Perspect* 1999;107(11):A556–560.
32. Tucker DA. Health care providers riding the information superhighway. *Home Care Providers* 1998;3(5):246–248.
33. Yoo T, Hut BY, Jean H, and Yun YH. Home telecare system integrated with periodic health reminder and medical record and multimedia health information. *Medinfo* 1998;9(pt 1):265–268.
34. Harris G. The new telecare: emerging Internet-based models for home healthcare. *Telemed Today* 1999;7(4):15–16.
35. London JW, Morton D, Marinucci D, Catalano R, and Comis RL. Cost effective Internet access and video conferencing for a community cancer network. *Proc Annu Symp Comput Appl Med Care* 1995;781–784.
36. Nagata H, Mizushima H. World wide microscope: new concept of internet telepathology microscope and implementation of the prototype. *Medinfo* 1998;9(pt 1):286–289.
37. McDonald CJ, Overstage JM, Tierney WM, et al. The Regenstrief Medical Record System: a quarter century experience. *Int J Med Inf* 1999;54(3):225–253.
38. Chin HL, Krall MA. Successful implementation of a comprehensive computer-based patient record system in Kaiser Permanente Northwest: strategy and experience. *Effect Clin Pract* 1998;1(2):51–60.
39. Shortliffe EH. The evolution of health-care records in the era of the Internet. *Medinfo* 1998;9(pt 1):8–14.
40. Shortliffe EH. The evolution of electronic medical records. *Acad Med* 1999;74(4): 414–419.
41. Rind DM, Kohane IS, Szolovits P, Safran C, Chue HC, and Barrett C. Maintaining the confidentiality of medical records shared over the Internet and the World Wide Web [see comments]. *Ann Intern Med* 1997;127(2):138–141.
42. Coile RC, Jr. Challenges for physician executives in the millennium marketplace. *Physician Exec* 1999;25(1):8–13.

7
Older Adults, Information Technology, and Behavioral Health Care

RAYMOND L. OWNBY, SARA J. CZAJA, AND CHIN CHIN LEE

Emerging information technologies are likely to have a significant impact on behavioral health care for the older adult. These technologies will provide improved access to information about mental health problems and their treatments. These improved information flows will allow for enhanced access to treatment services, and may even create new modes of service delivery for older patients. Current research shows that many older adults are interested in and willing to use information technologies, thus demonstrating the potential impact of information technologies in behavioral health care. Difficulties may arise, however, because problems with interface design and information architecture can create barriers to elderly patients' use of these technologies.

One of the most important aspects of information technologies, the Internet, is used by the elderly to access information about health care, community services and resources, and continuing education opportunities through the World Wide Web (WWW). The Internet can also be used to make routine tasks, such as financial management and shopping, easier. Access to these resources and services may be especially helpful to older people whose mobility is reduced or who have limited access to transportation. E-mail, however, is a key use of the Internet by many of the elderly.

Several studies have shown that older adults welcome opportunities to use e-mail and that its use increases social interactions among the elderly.[1,2] Galliene et al[3] found that access to a particular computer network, Computer-Link, augmented psychological support provided by nurses to homebound caregivers of patients with Alzheimer's disease. The computer network allowed these caregivers to access a support network to share experiences and develop new friendships.

Other studies support the observation that Internet applications are useful to the elderly. A study conducted by SeniorNet and Charles Schwab[4] showed that the Internet functions most often accessed by older adults are (1) exchanging e-mail with family and friends (72%), (2) researching a particular issue or subject (59%), (3) accessing news or current events (53%), (4) researching vacation or travel destination (47%), and (5) accessing local or regional weather information (43%). The study also indicates that the Web sites visited regularly among older adults are search engine Web sites (55%), news or current events sites (52%), hobby-specific sites (41%), health-related sites (39%), and investment sites (38%).

A more recent survey sponsored by the American Association of Retired Persons[5] illustrated similar patterns of computer use among older adults. In a sample of more than 1,000 computers users older than 45 years, 81% used their computers to access the Internet. E-mail was the most common reason for Internet access, with 90% using it for this purpose. Other common uses of the Internet included searching for information about products or services (73%), education (55%), chatting interactively (46%) and accessing healthcare information (42%).

Older adults clearly find information technologies such as the Internet valuable, and are willing to use them. A number of studies, however, show that although older people are interested in and are able to use information technologies such as Internet-connected computers, they often encounter greater obstacles to their use than do younger adults.[6,7] This chapter reviews a number of issues pertinent to the use of information technologies by older adults. The intent is to highlight the implications of age-related changes in perceptual and cognitive abilities for interface and information design. Before the full benefits of these types of technology can be realized from the elderly's perspective, it will be critically important that those who create healthcare information applications understand how to make them useful and usable by older adults. It is hoped is that this chapter will increase the awareness of older adults with specific needs as a population that should be addressed when developing information technology applications.

A central problem for Internet users is efficiently finding desired information. One survey of Internet users by the Georgia Institute of Technology Graphic, Visualization, and Usability Center in 1996 found that their most common problems were finding specific information, finding Web pages already visited, and slow Internet response time. At present, there are no standards systematically applied to the design of Web interfaces. This creates a number of usability problems, several of which are outlined by Vora and Helander[8]: outdated or incomplete information, poor use of graphics, slow response time, crowding information on the screen, and poor user navigation support. These problems are likely to worsen with the continuing expansion of the Web and the increasing number of Internet users. Finding information on the Web is often difficult and cumbersome, although indexes and search engines may help. For older adults, the problems are of even greater significance compared to younger persons. For example, decreased capacity in working memory among older adults may mean that poor navigational structures in a Web site may have a greater impact on them than the same problems in a younger counterpart.

Use of the Internet at its most basic level involves information seeking, a process that older adults undertake to find information or solve a problem. Information seeking is a high-level cognitive activity that encompasses a number of elemental cognitive processes, including memory, reasoning, attention, learning, and problem solving. Internet users develop information-seeking skills and strategies according to their abilities, experiences, and physical resources, such as information systems. Information seeking can be understood to be a process that results from the interaction among six factors: the information seeker, task, search system, information domain, setting, and search outcomes. The process can be both opportunistic and systematic and involves a number of interdependent subprocesses:

1. *Defining and understanding the problem:* Understanding the problem depends on knowledge of the task domain and may be influenced by the setting. For example, older adults' search for information about treatments for depression is inevitably influenced by their knowledge of depression and how it is treated.
2. *Formulation of a query:* Query formulation involves aligning the search task with the desired information system. In most cases, the initial query allows entry into the information system and is then followed by browsing or refinements of the initial query formulation. The older adult searching for information on depression might formulate the search by entering key words in a search engine or by going to a favorite health information site.
3. *Execution of the search:* Executing the physical actions for querying the information source is driven by the user's mental model of the search system. Users actually perform the search based on their physical interactions with the system. On the Internet, this means entering particular search terms or using the mouse to navigate to a specific Web site.
4. *Examination of results:* A query's execution leads to a result that needs user examination to validate result relevance with respect to the information-seeking task. For example, searching for information on depression might yield a variety of sites about various psychotherapeutic approaches, commercial sites touting herbal remedies, consumer self-help sites, and authoritative medical sites.
5. *Extraction of information:* Relevance assessments initiate actions for the extraction of information. When information is extracted, it is manipulated and integrated into the user's knowledge of the domain. The searcher evaluates various Web sites and chooses the one that seems most relevant to the query.
6. *Reflect/iterate/stop:* An information search is seldom complete with only a single query and retrieval. Deciding when and how to stop requires an assessment of the information-seeking process. Monitoring the information-seeking progress is crucial to the development of information seeking strategies.[9] For example, the searcher might evaluate information on several Web sites and then return to the search results page or a page of links before searching further. The searcher evaluates information at each step of the process, eventually deciding when to discontinue the search.

People develop strategies to guide the information-seeking process through practice and experience. This includes strategies for choosing and then searching information sources. As discussed by Marchionini,[9] information technologies like the Internet have had a dramatic impact on the process of information seeking. For example, instead of using a library and accessing hardcopy information, we now use on-line databases and access information in electronic form.

Information technologies, such as the Internet, require the information seeker to develop specialized knowledge and skills, including domain, system, and information-seeking expertise. *Domain expertise* helps seekers access information quickly and effectively. Experts in a domain usually have extensive topical knowledge and have it organized in a way that allows them to access it efficiently. *System expertise* refers to the knowledge and skills need for using the search system and its physical interface. In the case of the Internet, this includes the ability to use the keyboard, mouse, menus, windows, and computer screen. It also implies an understanding of how database documents are structured, database organization, and information availability. *Information-seeking expertise* refers to knowledge about and skills related to the very process of seeking information. This includes knowledge of relevant information sources and their organization. It also involves knowing where to look for information and then how to request it.

Information seeking is a highly variable process and individuals use strategies that vary according to task, context, and setting. Two broad categories can be distinguished: analytic and browsing. Analytic strategies are goal driven, and require precise and systematic planning methods that tend to be methodical and deterministic in nature. Browsing strategies are less methodical and are instead more opportunistic, informal, and interactive. Most people use a combination of analytic and browsing strategies when searching the WWW, but novice users and users with limited domain or system expertise are more likely to adopt browsing, rather than analytic, search strategies.[9] Browsing may result in chance discoveries and incidental learning, but can also result in the confusion, frustration, and cognitive overload that have been collectively referred to as being "lost in hyperspace."[10] Many older adults, when first approaching the Internet, have not had the opportunity to develop the expertise needed for efficient use of the current Internet search systems. Internet use for them requires learning a new set of skills for locating, accessing, manipulating, and utilizing information sources. Since increasing age is associated with decline in certain cognitive abilities, older adults may have greater difficulty in acquiring information search skills than younger adults.

Learning to use the Internet for communication and information thus may be a challenge for older adults. A number of studies have examined the older adult's ability to learn how to use information technologies. These studies have focused on diverse computer applications, like spreadsheets or word processors. Studies have also examined the effectiveness of different training strategies, such as conceptual versus procedural training[11] or computer- or instructor-based versus manual-based training.[12] The influence of other variables on learning, such as attitude toward computers and computer anxiety, has also been examined. Study results clearly show that older adults are able to use computers and information applications, but often have more difficulty in acquiring computer skills. In short, older adults ultimately require more training to acquire the same level of skills as younger people.

Egan and Gomez[13] conducted a series of experiments to identify the individual differences that would predict older adults' ability to learn text editing. Age and spatial memory were significant predictors of learning ability, with both variables contributing to predicting the number of first-try errors and time needed per successful edit. A greater age was associated with increased difficulty in producing the sequence of symbols needed to accomplish the desired edits.

Elias et al[14] studied age differences in the acquisition of text-editing skills, and identified the difficulties associated with skill acquisition in older adults. Training methods included an audiotape and a training manual. All participants were able to learn the fundamentals of word processing regardless of age, but the older adults required more time and help to complete the training program. Older adults also performed more poorly on a review examination. Garfein et al[15] examined the older adults' ability to learn how to use a spreadsheet. They also attempted to identify component abilities that would predict how well computer novices would acquire computer skills. All participants were able to operate the computer and use the spreadsheet package after two 90-minute training sessions. Fluid intelligence was an important predictor of performance, although significant age effects on performance were not found. This may have been because the age range of the participants was restricted to 49 to 67 years.

Gist et al[16] examined the influence of age and training method on acquiring spreadsheet-using skills. Training was either through a tutorial program or by behavioral modeling. In the tutorial approach, learners were provided with a computer-based step-by-step interactive instructional package. In the behavioral modeling approach, learners watched a videotape of a middle-aged man demonstrating the software and then practiced the procedure themselves. Both younger and older participants found the modeling approach to be superior to the tutorial, but the older adults performed more poorly on a posttraining test.

Zandri and Charness[17] investigated the influence of training method on older people's ability to use a calendar and notepad system, and examined whether providing an advanced organizer would have an impact on the acquisition of computer skills in younger and older adults. They also studied whether or not learning with a partner would influence skill acquisition. Their results demonstrated interactions among age, training method (alone or with a peer), organizer (with or without), and performance. For older adults who trained without a partner, the use of an advanced organizer resulted in better performance. For the other older adults, no effect on performance was observed. For younger subjects, the use of an advanced organizer resulted in worse performance if they learned alone but made no difference if they learned with a partner. These results suggest that an advanced organizer may have different effects on learning for older people. Older people were about 2.5 times slower than their younger counterparts in the training sessions, and required about three times as much as help.

In a follow-up study, Charness et al[18] examined the impact of training techniques and computer anxiety on the acquisition of word processing skills in samples of younger and older adults. In the first portion of this study, 16 computer novices ranging in age from 25 to 81 learned word processing skills with a self-paced training program. Only half of the participants received an advanced organizer prior to training. The organizer did not appear to improve performance.

Older adults took about 1.2 times longer than the younger adults to complete training, and required more help. In the second part of the study, the investigators attempted to control the nature of the training session. Thirty computer novices were assigned to either a self-paced learning condition, where they became actively involved in the tutorial, or a fixed-paced condition, where they passively observed a predetermined sequence of activities. The younger and older adults both performed better in the self-paced training condition, although the older adults again took nearly 1.2 times longer to complete training and required more help.

Czaja et al[12] evaluated three novice adult training strategies for learning to use a word processing program. The training strategies were instructor-, manual-, and on-line training-based. Younger adults were more successful in learning the word processing program than the older adults, who were slower and made more errors. The manual- and instructor-based training were superior to on-line training for all participants. The investigators found age differences in performance on posttraining tasks, with older adults making more errors and taking more time to complete tasks.

In another study, Czaja et al[19] attempted to identify a training strategy in learning text editing that would minimize age differences. Two training programs were evaluated: a goal-oriented program and a traditional approach that included a manual and lecture. The goal-oriented approach introduced the elements of text editing in an incremental fashion, moving from simple to more complex tasks. The training sessions included problem-solving tasks with the objectives of discovering and achieving methods for completing them. The manual was written as a series of goal-oriented units, and used simple language. Similarities were drawn between computers and familiar concepts, and the amount of necessary reading was kept to a minimum. Participants who were trained with the goal-oriented approach had better posttraining performance; these participants took less time to complete the tasks and made fewer mistakes. In spite of manipulating the training method, older adults' performances were still worse than their younger cohorts. Older adults required more time to complete tasks, completed fewer editing changes, and made more mistakes.

Caplan and Schooler[20] evaluated whether or not providing the participants with a conceptual model of the software would improve their ability to learn a painting software program. They provided half of the participants with an analogical model of the program before training. Results indicated that the model was beneficial for the younger adults but was detrimental to the older adults. Similar results were found by Morrell et al.[11] They studied the ability of young-old (ages 60 to 74 years) and old-old (ages 75 to 89) adults to perform tasks on ELDER-COMM, a computer bulletin board system. Participants were presented with either procedural instructions alone or a combination of conceptual information and procedural instructions. All participants performed better with the procedural instruction-only material. Young-old adults performed better than the old-old adults, as the old-old adults made more performance errors. The investigator concluded that conceptual training might not have benefited the older adults because they needed to translate the model into action, and that this additional process may have increased the task's working memory demands.

In summary, research has shown that older adults are able to use computers for routine tasks and are able to learn a wide variety of computer applications. They are usually slower at acquiring computer skills than younger adults and require more help and hands-on practice to acquire similar levels of skill. Older adults often require additional training in basic computer skills, such as using the mouse or managing windows, when training in a particular computer application. They may also require information on the types of available technologies, the potential benefits associated with using these technologies, and where and how to access them. Finally, greater attention needs to be given to training and instructional materials design in order to accommodate age-related changes in perceptual and cognitive abilities.

As discussed earlier, information seeking is a complex process and places demands on a number of cognitive abilities such as working and spatial memory, reasoning, and problem solving. Information seeking within an electronic environment also requires skills specific to that environment, such as knowledge related to the search system or its interface. Older adults often experience declines in certain cognitive abilities, such as working memory, and are less likely than younger people to have knowledge of the structure and organization of search systems. A relevant question to ask is this: To what degree will they have trouble when searching for information in an electronic environment? Although the topic of electronic information search and retrieval has received considerable attention within the human-computer interaction literature, the available data for older people on this topic is limited.

Westerman et al[21] examined the relationship between spatial ability, spatial memory, vocabulary skills, age, and the ability to retrieve information from a computer database that varied according to how the database was structured (hierarchical versus linear). Older participants retrieved information more slowly than the younger adults did; however, the researchers did not find age-related differences in accuracy. Learning rates differed between the two groups, with the older participants learning more slowly than the younger participants. The slower response speed among the older adults was more dependent on general processing speed than on other cognitive abilities.

Freudenthal[22] examined the extent to which response latencies in an information retrieval task were predicted by movement speed and other cognitive variables within a group of younger and of older adults. Participants were required to search for answers in a hierarchical menu structure. Older participants had longer overall latencies for information retrieval than younger participants, and these latencies increased with each of the menu's steps. Similar to Westerman et al,[21] Freudenthal found that movement speed was a significant predictor of overall latency and that other cognitive abilities, such as reasoning speed, spatial ability, and memory, also predicted response latencies. Memory and spatial abilities were only predictors for latency on deeper steps in the menu structure. Freudenthal suggests that deep menu structures may not be appropriate for older adults, as navigation through these types of structures is dependent on spatial skills that tend to decline with age. Vicente et al[23] also found that age, spatial ability, and vocabulary predicted search latencies in a computer information retrieval task. They suggested that people with low spatial ability tended to become lost while searching the database. Other investigators such as Gomez et al,[24] Sein and Bostrom,[25] and Czaja and Sharit[6] have also discovered that spatial ability predicts performance on computer-interactive tasks.

Mead et al[26] examined younger and older adults' ability to use an on-line library database. Younger adults were more successful than older adults in performing the searches, and used more efficient search strategies. Older adults made more errors in formulating search queries and had greater difficulty in recovering from their errors. A study by Czaja and Sharit[27] examined age differences in a database inquiry task. The task was a simulation of a customer service representative's assignment in the health insurance industry. Participants were required to search through computerized data files to answer "customer" questions about their health insurance coverage. Older adults completed fewer queries and were less effective in documenting their responses, but no age differences in navigational efficiency were found after accounting for differences in response speed. Age, cognitive abilities such as working memory and spatial skills, and prior computer experience also influenced performance. Prior experience with computers was an important predictor of performance, as were cognitive abilities such as working memory and processing speed. As expected, older participants had less prior experience with computers than did the younger participants. Czaja and Sharit suggest that providing older adults with basic computer training is as important as providing them with application training. Results for all participants also proved that performance improved with task experience. This finding reinforces the importance of providing older adults with adequate training and opportunities for practicing novel skills.

In a study of the how the elderly search the World Wide Web, Mead et al[7] found that older adults used less efficient search strategies and were less successful than the younger adults in searching the Web for specific information. Older people often had difficulty remembering previously followed links and information on previously searched pages. The data suggest that history markers may be of particular benefit to older people.

In summary, available research shows that older adults have the ability to search and retrieve information in electronic environments that are typical of information technology applications. Older adults tend to use less efficient navigation strategies and have more difficulty with search and retrieval tasks than do younger adults. They have greater difficulty in remembering where and what they are searching for. To maximize older people's ability to successfully interact with electronic information systems such as the WWW and access the information superhighway, we need to have an understanding of age-related difficulties. This information will allow us to develop interfaces and training strategies that will accommodate individual differences in performance. There is currently very little information on problems experienced by older adults as they learn to navigate the Web, especially in the context of the real world. Additional research will be an important prerequisite in making behavioral healthcare information technologies more readily accessible to older adults.

References

1. Furlong MS. An electronic community for older adults: the SeniorNet network. *J Commun* 1989;39:145–153.
2. Czaja SJ, Guerrier J, Nair S, Laudauer T. Computer communication as an aid to independence for older adults. *Behav Information Technol* 1993;2:97–107.
3. Galliene RL, Moore SM, Brennan PF. Alzheimer's caregivers: psychosocial support via computer network. *J Gerontol Nurs* 1993;12:1–22.
4. SeniorNet and Charles Schwab. *Graying of the Internet,* 1998 (On-line). *http://www. headcount.com/globalsource/profile/index.htm?choice=ussenior&id=190.*
5. American Association of Retired Persons. AARP National Survey on Consumer Preparedness and E-Commerce: a survey of computer users age 45 and older (on-line). *http://research.aarp.org/consume/ecommerce_1.html*
6. Czaja SJ, Sharit J. Ability-performance relationships as a function of age and task experience for a data entry task. *J Exp Psychol Appl* 1998;4:332–351.
7. Mead SE, Spaulding VA, Sit RA, Meyer B, Walker N. Effects of age and training on World Wide Web navigation strategies. *Proceedings of the Human Factors and Ergonomics Society, 41st annual meeting.* Albuerquerque, NM. 1997:152–156.
8. Vora PR, Helander MG. Hypertex and its implications for the Internet. In: Helander MG, Landauer TK, Prabhu PV, eds. *Handbook of Human-Computer Interaction,* 2nd ed. Amsterdam, The Netherlands: Elsevier, 1997:877–914.
9. Marchionini G. *Information Seeking in Electronic Environments.* Cambridge, UK: Cambridge University Press, 1995.
10. Nielsen J. *Hypertext and hypermedia.* Boston: Academic Press, 1990.
11. Morrell RW, Park DC, Mayhorn CB, Echt KV. Older adults and electronic communication networks: learning to use ELDERCOMM. Paper presented at the 103rd annual convention of the American Psychological Association, New York, 1995.
12. Czaja SJ, Hammond K, Blascovich J, Swede H. Age-related differences in learning to use a text-editing system. *Behav Information Technol* 1989;8:309–319.
13. Egan DE, Gomez LM. Assaying, isolating, and accommodating individual differences in learning a complex skill. *Individual Differ Cogn* 1985;2:174–217.
14. Elias PK, Elias MF, Robbins MA, Gage P. Acquisition of word-processing skills by younger, middle-aged, and older adults. *Psychol Aging* 1987;2:340–348.
15. Garfein AJ, Schaie KW, Willis SL. Microcomputer proficiency in later-middle-aged adults and older adults: teaching old dogs new tricks. *Social Behav* 1988;3:131–148.
16. Gist M, Rosen B, Schwoerer C. The influence of training method and trainee age on the acquisition of computer skills. *Personal Psychol* 1988;41:255–265.
17. Zandri E, Charness N. Training older and younger adults to use software. *Educ Gerontol* 1989;15:615–631.
18. Charness N, Schumann CE, Boritz GA. Training older adults in word processing: effects of age, training technique and computer anxiety. *Int J Aging Technol* 1992;5:79–106.
19. Czaja SJ, Hammond K, Joyce JB. Word processing training for older adults. Final report submitted to the National Institute on Aging. Grant # 5 R4 AGO4647-03, 1989.

20. Caplan LJ, Schooler C. The effects of analogical training models and age on problem solving in a new domain. *Exp Aging Res* 1990;16:151–154.
21. Westerman SJ, Davies DR, Glendon AI, Stammer RB, Matthews G. Age and cognitive ability as predictors of computerized information retrieval. *Behav Information Technol* 1995;14:313–326.
22. Freudenthal D. Learning to use interactive devices; age differences in the reasoning process. Master's thesis, Eindhoven University of Technology, 1997.
23. Vicente KJ, Hayes BC, Williges RC. Assaying and isolating individual differences in searching a hierarchical file system. *Hum Factors* 1987;29:349–359.
24. Gomez LM, Egan DE, Wheeler EA, Sharma DK, Gruchacz AM. How interface design determines who had difficulty learning to use a text editor. *Proceedings of the CHI 83 Conferences on Human Factors in Computer Systems*. Boston, MA. 1983:176–181.
25. Sein MK, Bostrom RP. Individual differences in conceptual models in training novice users. *Hum Comput Interaction* 1989;4:197–229.
26. Mead SE, Sit RA, Jamieson BA, Rousseau GK, Rogers WA. Online library catalog: age-related differences in performance for novice users. Paper presented at the annual meeting of the American Psychological Association, Toronto, Canada, 1996.
27. Czaja SJ, Sharit J. Age differences in a complex information search and retrieval task. Annual meeting of the American Psychological Association, Boston, 1999.

Part IV
Informatics and
Quality Improvement

Introduction

WILLIAM S. EDELL

There has been a remarkable transformation in behavioral health care over the last 20 years that cannot be overstated. What was once believed to be impossible is now held to be imperative. The notion that one can, and indeed must, quantify psychological phenomena in a meaningful and actionable framework to demonstrate quality and justify reimbursement is no longer questioned. Indeed, the careful measurement of outcomes, broadly defined to include clinical, economic, and humanistic domains, using well-designed, psychometrically sound instruments, is now understood to be essential to survive and thrive in the highly competitive marketplace.

Our society has concurrently experienced unparalleled information technology growth. How could any graduate student of the late 1970s forget lugging boxes of computer cards through the snow to the university computer center to insert them into metal card readers attached to massive computers, and then on a good day wait for output in a bin 15 minutes later? Small errors could extend the waiting time into hours or days. In addition, report writing meant spending days or weeks in the library poring over books and articles—if they were not checked out or missing from the shelves. In contrast, students today can research the world's literature on any topic of interest and can instantaneously obtain newly published reports from the comfort of their home, at any time convenient to them. For those not fortunate to have a personal computer of their own, public libraries afford free and easy access to the World Wide Web. The newer information technologies explosion is likely to transform our world further, specifically health care, in ways we can only begin to imagine. It seems clear that educated consumers and their families will no longer tolerate healthcare providers who are not similarly staying abreast of the latest treatments for their condition. Neither will payers seek to do business with those not genuinely committed to providing the very best treatments for producing the very best outcomes, all in a cost-efficient manner.

How best to link the exciting developments in quality improvement with those in behavioral healthcare information technology is the focus of the chapters in this section. Although coming from distinct sectors of the healthcare environment (managed care and the government), they provoke the reader to consider both the enormous power and responsibilities involved in such associations. It is important to emphasize that not all information is necessarily accurate or true. The notion that "more is better" may be true for a research scientist doing a meta-analysis of an extensive literature, but the average consumer may feel lost and overwhelmed in the proverbial "forest for the trees" without guidance and training in just *how* to understand and use the information presented.

There is an enormous need for continued thoughtful, sensitive, and intelligent discussion on how best to define such terms as *good outcome*, *provider competence*, and *high quality* in behavioral health care. Those of us who have toiled in these fields for many years understand the underlying complexity of these expressions, and that the answers will come not from the simple and mindless accumulation of information and quality improvement projects. Instead, they will come from the accrued wisdom of the many players (consumers, families, providers, and payers, to name a few) involved in the behavioral healthcare environment.

8
Managing Clinical Care in a Pervasive Computing Environment

Les DelPizzo, Sarbori R. Bhattacharya, Naakesh A. Dewan, and Suresh Bangara

Behavioral health care is, for the most part, an information-driven activity. In fact, it is possible to view the caregiving transaction as an exchange of information. This chapter discusses technology issues related to the electronic capture, dissemination, and analysis of clinical information. Each of these processes involves a combination of factors, including emerging, but immature, technology. One must consider the shrinking resource base for private practitioners and organized providers, thus limiting the capital needed to invest in technology. Finally, there is a lack of a critical mass of appropriate technology spread throughout the behavioral health industry. Each of these processes represents distinct challenges, in terms of applying information technology.

The desktop computer may not be the weapon of choice in this real-time, "need-it-now" environment. Desktop computing succumbs to pervasive computing. IBM uses the term *pervasive computing* to define a significant segment of its ongoing research and product development. Information technology (IT) industry periodicals tout this concept as "the next big thing" until, of course, the *next* next big thing appears. The National Institute of Standards and Technology (NIST), however, looks beyond hype. Instead, NIST sponsors conferences and convenes groups to create standards for this emerging technology; any subject that is the topic of a government-sponsored event has duly passed from "cutting edge" to mainstream.

NIST defines pervasive computing as

shorthand for the strongly emerging trend toward:

- Numerous, casually accessible, often invisible computing devices
- Frequently mobile or imbedded in the environment
- Connected to an increasingly ubiquitous network structure

The aim is for easier computing, more available everywhere it's needed.

Because "pervasive computing" so succinctly captures the blending of technologies and the goal of "wherever, whenever, however" computing, it is important to fully explore the implications of this definition.

Information Flow Dilemma in Contemporary Health Care

A major duty of the healthcare professional is to assess the information gleaned from the client and others, and then use that information to collaborate with the client in some health-enhancing way. Accreditation and/or state licensing requirements, operating on the "If it isn't written, it didn't happen" principle, require documentation of any client/patient and caregiver information, thus giving rise to the phenomenon known as "paperwork." Paperwork, to a clinician, is time spent interacting with paper instead of clients. Turn it into an electronic process, and clinicians would still consider it "paperwork" since it is *about* clients, not *with* clients. Clinicians are drowning in paperwork because of the client documentation requirements demanded by major payers. Major payers require proof of medical necessity, a clinical concept requiring clinical judgment couched in clinical terms, as well as proof of value. Proving value requires some clinical or functional definition of desired outcome.

This information flow is now more critical than ever. Information is passed from the client through the practitioner to others in the healthcare organization. This then is sent to external parties, primarily the payers of the client's healthcare services, thus directly impacting the practitioner's viability, whether that practitioner is an individual or an organization. When Medicare demands millions of dollars back from hospitals and community mental health centers, primarily because treatment records could not support billings, the need to control that clinical information flow becomes a matter of fiduciary survival, not simply a matter of best practice.

Information flows within the behavioral healthcare industry have changed in quantity and quality, impacted by the previously noted factors:

• Payers have migrated more risk to providers or other intermediary organizations.
• Providers must meet an expanding variety of licensing and accreditation expectations.
• Value is now the defining criterion for success in the marketplace.

Prior to the impact of the factors noted above, clinicians simply had to report the type of service, the length of treatment, and information regarding the recipient. Due to these factors, they now had to document a plethora of information that flows from the client's eligibility for service. This included problems faced by the client, thus creating a need for service, the lowest level of service required to meet this need, the interventions used as part of the service, and their resulting outcomes. This information overload inundated all paper-based systems, rendering them useless. For the sake of the chapter, let us call this era the "tsunami period." Equally important, this vast volume of information represented data of a completely different type than previously collected. Thus, both volume and type are compelling disrupters to clinical care.

As providers took on more financial risk and were required to document every aspect of the patient–provider interaction, they realized that they needed to answer different, more complex questions:

• How can they define the client's problem so that they simultaneously outline the level of care to be provided?
• How can the activities of multiple practitioners be coordinated to create an optimal intervention episode for the client, so that the least amount of resources are used to meet the need, and the client derives the highest level of satisfaction from the episode?
• How can the provider of the services convey the value of the services to the payer, as well as to future and current clients?

Confronted with such questions, the practitioners learned that their practice management systems were unable to satisfy them, since their systems were never created to answer such questions. These particular questions require the integration of clinical information with financial, demographic, and administrative data, thus needing the generation, dissemination, and analysis of clinical information in order to answer them.

Historically, healthcare providers had adopted information technology primarily to handle their business operations; few clinics or healthcare offices lacked computers on the desks of the administration, receptionist, and back office billing. Driven by event data—who did what to whom and for what period of time—these back-office systems adequately handled fee-for-service billing. Institutional providers could expect more from their automated practice management systems, such as accounts payable, budget, payroll, and inventory management, but all of these functions are essentially back-office activities. Most private practitioners would, even now, describe it as state-of-the-art practice management if one were to add scheduling to the current system.

Disillusioned by their overwhelming paper systems, clinicians turned to their computer-based system, expecting it to be their productivity solution. However, as noted earlier, these systems, essentially back-office in nature, were never created to meet such expectations. Capturing clinical data electronically is challenging for at least two reasons: clinicians in the past have never had to capture such great volumes of highly complex information. Second, capturing clinical data requires the integration of a broad range of technologies, all of which are in an emerging state. In the face of the overwhelming need to create and capture information, one would expect a virtual blossoming of the informatics market, with clinicians using technology to capture clinical information faster, cheaper, better. Unfortunately, disappointments abound. After all, few clinicians, especially in organized settings, have a computer on their desk, and those who do find that it meets only a limited number of their needs. This void can be explained by a combination of the following factors:

• emerging, but immature, technology
• a shortage of appropriate technology within the behavioral health industry

• a shrinking resource base for private practitioners and organized providers, limiting the capital needed to invest in technology.

This chapter expands upon the above factors and deals with technology issues that are related to the electronic capture, dissemination, and analysis of clinical information. Each of these processes represents distinct challenges, with respect to applying information technology. Each of these processes must be technologically harnessed for clinicians to answer the questions posed earlier.

A Primer on Data Capture

As previously mentioned, clinicians are now required to capture a greater volume of complex information than ever before. To get a sense of the new requirements, it is crucial to remember that the electronic world is a binary one. All information in the electronic world must be coded, or translated, from the multivariate world into a binary one. The process of coding is complex and arduous, and people in the field avoid it, if given a choice. Next, the very act of capturing this clinical data requires the integration of a broad range of technologies, all of which are in their infancy.

Coding comes in many forms. One such form is *software*, or coding that mediates transactions between the physical and binary worlds. We then create categories of information, represented by numbers or letters that are easily input, or entered, into the software. Because of the complexity of the process, we welcome *standards*, or codes that come to mean the same thing to those who regularly deal with the code information.

Before the tsunami period, the information and standard codes used were broadly derived. The back-office, computer-based systems both created and depended on these codes. Because the billing system was of primary importance, standard-coding systems evolved to define provider services, namely the current procedure terminology (CPT) codes. Standard billing forms, such as the UB 92 and HCFA 1500, evolved around where to place standard codes. All other required elements, such as the service providers and their credentials, the service recipient (reduced to a number), and the duration of service, were easily coded. As this coded infrastructure developed over time, the software, which translated these standard codes into the binary reality that hardware could process, also developed in power and sophistication. Information technology could now easily absorb the data, although the process of applying information technology to information processes required congruence between the technology used and the coding of the information. These processes were interdependent; neither was sufficient on its own.

This pre-tsunami world was batch-oriented in nature. Entered data did not have to be accessed in real time. Bills could be run at periodic times, dictated only by volume and cash flow needs. Other information, such as budgets, vendor payments, and provider productivity, could also be bundled into reports that were periodically created and used. In short, there was a discontinuity between data capture and data processing. Given the parameters of this period, however, that discontinuity reflected its requirements. Clinical information was electronically irrelevant; it existed in the carbon paper world.

The contrast with the post-tsunami world is stunning. Because there was no history of collecting behavioral healthcare clinical information, no group of software applications reflected how clinicians actually worked and integrated clinical with financial and administrative data. Behavioral healthcare clinical practice was subdivided into multiple, often warring, disciplines that had different "schools of practice" within each discipline. These subdivisions often created sharper disagreements than those of the parents. Other than the *Diagnostic and Statistical Manual of Mental Disorders* (DSM), which codified behavioral health diagnoses, there was no set of universally accepted clinical protocols; practitioners did not follow a standard practice. Thus, there was no coding infrastructure available to categorize clinical information. In the absence of any standard content that could be coded into software, there was no broadly accepted software available for clinical processes.

Niche systems existed at one time and will continue to do so. These software packages generally automated only one aspect of the clinical process, such as treatment planning, or specific assessment instruments. In no case, however, did these software applications integrate into practice management applications. There was no way to provide for the comprehensive data stream required to meet the new demands.

Other elements of the clinical information flow reflected the same segmentation. Eligibility for service varied from contract to contract. No universal menu of benefits existed, as risk-managing enterprises used the benefit plan as a marketing differential. The administrative risk manager defined "medical necessity." Value was not measured by standard outcomes.

Integration of Multiple, Emerging Technologies

The exchange of clinical information between a clinician and consumer is separate from the information transaction that occurs between the clinician and technology. Bridging this gap is what pervasive computing is all about.

Before we explore further the conditions required for technology and clinical transactions, we need to explore some of the implications of such an action. The first issue is that this post-tsunami world is a real-time, as opposed to a "batch-oriented," world. As clinical and technology transactions co-occur, entered data will determine what additional information needs to be captured and what care might be appropriate. This will happen in real time, as the clinician works with the client.

As part of the intake process, for example, there are usually questions that attempt to assess the risk the client poses to himself or to others. In our envisioned electronic world, different responses to the question about suicidal thoughts would generate different follow-up questions. A "no" would be followed by a question about suicide history. The patient can answer with different levels of "yes," such as "Yes, but not in the last 3 months" as opposed to "Yes, in the last 24 hours." The resulting answer presents different questions for the clinician to act upon, such as ask and answer, probe for intent, level of plan, and access to means. Equally important, these answers shape the approach to intervention, presenting the clinician with prelisted problem areas to address upon beginning the treatment plan. Health severity indicators are being developed to facilitate level-of-care decisions (IHP Corp., Seattle, Washington, 1999).

In this real-time world, the content of software applications will drive the merging of reporting and intervention practice. We are establishing the technologies and skill base required to develop, maintain, and enhance such content in our efforts at "knowledge management." We are only now starting to master the art of creating this type of comprehensive, multiuse clinical content. The "art," in this case, is in creating a rich universe of data points that captures the clinical processes and workflow actually used by clinicians. The more we capture the intervention with data points, the more downstream leverage we exert, since these data points can be used for so many complementary purposes.

Data points can be transformed from real time to narrative reports. In fact, these data points can be converted into a broad range of reports, so that a single effort on the clinician's part can result in the completion of multiple tasks. For example, upon finishing an electronic intake that embeds carefully developed clinical content, a clinician can

- print out a report in a format approved by her agency for inclusion in the paper record,
- print out or review and then electronically send a medical necessity report to the behavioral health risk manager,
- digitally sign and authenticate and then send a copy of the intake report to the client's electronic medical record, and
- send selected data points to the outcome data warehouse.

Rich clinical content, however, must consist of more than data points. Narration is needed to qualify, individualize, and create a context for the data points. While narrative statements are difficult to code and analyze, they are critical in capturing the richness of the clinical intervention. Some state licensing personnel, in fact, recoil from automated treatment plans because they view the outcome of such applications as "canned." Automated treatment plans are seen by some as incapable of making specific and individualizing connections among the intake process, treatment planning, and ongoing service documentation. Properly developed clinical content with spare, but leveraged, narrative text should strike a balance between data input simplicity for clinicians and rich, individualized data reporting.

There are technological implications associated with this reliance upon narrative text. Electronic speech-to-text capability will be critical to any technology that brings together reporting and intervention practice. The ability to quickly dictate, as opposed to typing, narrative text will greatly increase not only the clinicians' accessibility to, but also the acceptance of, informatics. It is important to note, however, that speech recognition technology has one severe limitation: it is best used *after* a face-to-face interaction with the client. Few clinicians would be so rude as to dictate narrative in the client's presence. Most of today's clinicians would prefer a paperwork-eliminating system, even if they had to use the precious time after direct client interactions to do the data capture. Unfortunately, the ideal situation from a productivity standpoint is for data capture to occur as the intervention occurs.

Assuming our industry is artful enough to create clinical content that actually reflects the clinicians' work, the technology that we use to deposit information would have to have other critical abilities. Static information becomes progressively useless since clinical protocols change. The practice of intervention itself would change as the result of systematic outcome analysis, as new evidence-based practice replaced or supplemented the old. Licensing and accreditation systems change, thus spurring reporting changes down to the client-practitioner level; state licensing and reporting requirements change significantly over time. Thus, the technology that embeds clinical content would have to include tools that enable clinicians to change the content as needed.

Another level of flexibility is also required. As noted earlier, one dimension of informatics is the push for "one-pass" productivity: the clinician's ability to complete multiple tasks with one pass of work. The ability to generate multiple reports with the same data points is at the heart of these multiple tasks. As compelling as this ability may be, its value is limited if there is no easy way to create and modify report formats. This capability is so important it embraces the theory that clinicians are willing to accept limited variability in the data input process, as long as they can create significant variability in the data reporting process. The reasons for this theory parallel those noted earlier: things change.

With the institution of content established, as well as the need to have tools that can create and modify it, we can now turn to the technologies required to embed this information. The important thing to remember is that a variety of technologies are involved and all must interrelate. To concentrate our review of technologies, we need to start with the clinicians. What are their expectations with regards to technology?

The Promise of Technology

One must consider several baseline expectations when developing clinical applications to meet clinicians' needs:

• Technology must reduce the amount of time spent on paperwork by operating on a true "single entry" process. Once entered, the information should be available without having to enter it again elsewhere in the intervention; it is simply provided by the system.

- The system should alert clinicians if they have done something patently foolish or could increase their own or their employer's risk.
- Technology should be transparent, nonintrusive, and intuitive. One should be able to use it effortlessly.
- Technology should not force clinicians to change their work patterns in order to accommodate it.

This last point warrants some additional attention. First, one should appreciate how clinicians work. Clinical activity does not occur in a vacuum; clinicians must take into account a variety of practical considerations. Clients must be scheduled for future interventions, which in turn must be filtered through authorizations for service. Clinicians must report to others how they use their time, especially for billing purposes. The expectation is that these supporting functions will be fully integrated into clinical applications. Quick, one-click access to a scheduling tool saves valuable time and reflects how clinicians want their work to flow. Rapid access to authorized services is invaluable when planning interventions. An option at the end of any reporting or documentation transaction should be the ability to record a clinician's time. This type of organically featured technology, coupled with the appropriate clinical content, begins to close the gap between reporting and intervention practice.

Turning to the "where" of intervention practice, a shrinking proportion of clinicians are desk-bound. In the public sector, the push to serve the most severely disabled has created a spate of services that have a rehabilitative approach and are delivered at scattered sites throughout the community. This is often called a "wraparound" service by clinicians, who borrowed the term from the children's services that describes this approach. Wraparound services are the antithesis of institutionally based services. Rather than place the person in a specialized environment, individualized services are provided, or "wrapped around," in the general environment—home, school, and the workplace. In both the private and public sector, highly skilled and appropriately credentialed staff periodically travel circuits that take them to multiple service locations. These may include satellite offices within their practices, nursing homes, hospitals, schools, and group homes. Inpatient and residential services require staff to move from room to room and floor to floor; even practitioners who do not provide wraparound services may work in a facility or campus that requires them to move about. All levels of staff, from physicians to aides, are mobile in such environments.

This high degree of mobility by an increasing number of behavioral healthcare staff means that any technology that seeks to converge reporting and intervention practice must be available anywhere, any time. Since the clinical transactions must be mobile, the reporting must be as well. The mobile staff requires more than reporting capacity; staff members must constantly access information in order to do their work. In this real-time world, clinical information comes as a constantly changing stream as providers intervene with the client. As we shall see later, the client may contribute to this stream of information independent of the practitioners, as health care becomes increasingly self-interventional in nature.

The conjunction of reporting and intervention practice depends on using a variety of tools: the desktop will not be supplanted; it will be supplemented. What are these tools? They range from existing popular personal data appliances (PDAs) such as the Palm Pilot to digital cell phones, and include technology often referred to as "wearable computers," which is only now being prototyped in labs around the world. The point is that we will be using a range of intensely focused bundles of technology made for very specific uses.

Companies will be introducing their plethora of appliances into an extremely competitive market. Thus, prices will tend to be low to moderate and will lead to these items quickly becoming commodities, just as most kitchen appliances are now. The pricing and wide availability will lead to technology that is "casually accessible." This phrase refers to more than price; it also refers to ease of use. Unlike the complex, general-purpose desktop computer, these appliances will be designed with simplicity of use in mind, with interfaces that make sense, either because, like the phone, we already know how to use them, or because they are designed to serve limited purposes for broad audiences. These appliances, in short, will be *cool*. As we all know, *cool* sells.

If low price and *cool* were not enough, it is quite possible that many of these appliances will be casually accessible because they are free, especially those with only basic functions. One way to get them into people's hands quickly and on a scale that makes a difference is to give them away. With a large enough market, such appliances can generate revenues by providing access to a large number of users. In such a model, the appliance becomes the medium for special advertising and for broadband network services.

Clinicians will easily adapt to these ubiquitous PDAs, especially as they mature in function. Case managers and wraparound staff will soon download information from their desktop computer into the PDA and then use it as a data input device as they make their circuit through client homes and other community locations. Clinical content will be artfully designed to require the clinician to simply "point and tap" entered data. Once returned to the office, the clinician can upload this information into the desktop computer. Programs residing on the desktop or a strategically placed server will use these data points to generate fully formatted paper and electronic medical records, and then send outcome data to the data warehouse. The upload and download will not be necessary as this technology matures, since the PDA will eventually talk directly to an omnipresent network.

A high degree of pervasiveness is implied by such a broad use of appliances, but they represent only the first layer. Any object onto which a silicon chip can be embedded is a potential computing device. We can see how pervasive these devices are in our society as soon as we disconnect ourselves from objects with any form of computing ability. Anything is capable of being an "invisible computing device"; recent reports in the technical press speak of chips that can be embedded onto anything printable. Bill Joy has already created a programming system, Jini, that easily and efficiently recognizes and manages these embedded computers. However unrealistic such capacities may seem now, they will eventually integrate into the healthcare staff's everyday work. A perfect example of this assimilation: an intravenous pouch that pages a staff member once it reaches a defined level of use, alerting the staff to replace it with a new one.

Connecting to an Increasingly Ubiquitous Network Structure

This network, of course, is the Internet and enterprise LANs and WANs built on Internet standards. Ubiquity will be maximized when these local and wide-area networks are wireless and when clinicians are finally removed from any physical connection to network services. Someday, the universal gateway to information will be an Internet browser, and all appliances, including cell phones, will be browser-enabled.

The rapid development of the wireless Internet provides the infrastructure for increasing network permeation. Presently, limited bandwidth and spotty coverage across broad geographical regions make wireless connectivity either a curiosity or a toy for technophiles. New standards and technologies, however, point to dramatic bandwidth increases and system interoperability. A perfect example is TeraBeam. This new start-up has already inked a deal with Lucent Technology to offer fiberless optic transmission, based on laser technology that reaches gigabit-per-second speeds. Such speeds are much higher than cable modems and DSL, the most common "last mile" technologies now in use. There has been increasing acceptance of the wireless application protocol (WAP) by a broad range of vendors for the pursuit of aggressive technology development while remaining confident that these technologies can be integrated into practical, value-adding systems.

Thus, it would appear that the future of behavioral healthcare informatics—the convergence of clinical and technology transactions—is to be defined by increasingly sophisticated clinical content embedded within a pervasive computing environment. There are, however, a number of impediments to this envisioned future. Ironically, one of the most significant happens to be technology-based: the security of networked clinical data.

Health care, and behavioral health care in particular, maintains that the highest value is placed on the *privacy* of individual information, even though the *security* of transmitted data is a major concern for all commercial networked enterprises. Healthcare practitioners and consumers must insist upon privacy, especially at a time when the definition of individual privacy on the public Web and on corporate intra- and extranets is one of the great public debates. The existence of medical privacy as a protected entity remains to be seen. The technology ensuring such privacy is slowly evolving, but it is critical to note that it is yet another set of emerging technologies that must mature before full use of a pervasive computing environment is appropriate for healthcare practitioners. Maturity, in this context, means transparency. Practitioners must trust nonintrusive and invisible technologies to provide the highest level of security and privacy possible.

Security is not the only obstacle faced by behavioral healthcare informatics. "Critical mass" is needed in the field prior to technology's making a difference. We can better understand this phenomenon by turning to an exploration of the second crucial clinical process—the dissemination, or sharing of, information.

Sharing Clinical Information: Leveraging Real-Time Communication

Clinicians may be motivated to use informatics since it can reduce the time they spend on paperwork; they can shift from a paper shuffling to a point-and-click accessibility. Once information is digitized, its value is not measured solely in the paper savings and unused physical space; it also lies in the ease of access and sharing. These additional benefits are important for two reasons. First, the value can be measured in the amount of time saved by clinicians' not having to root through vast quantities of physical documents. Second, worth can be measured by the increased quality derived from clinicians' having important information in real time, when and where they need it.

This second and most profound value, however, comes at a price. All clinicians in an enterprise have to be wired for this value to be obvious; they must *all* have access to the technology. At a minimum, there has to be some critical mass of clinicians using this informatics technology in order for sharing to take place. An analogy is fax machines, a stand-in for any two-node technology. Their use started as a trickle, since the utility of faxing was only apparent if others had fax machines. It was only when these machines became ever-present that the full value of the technology unfolded. To some extent, exactly the same dynamic characterizes healthcare informatics.

It would be a mistake, however, to view the creation of this critical mass of clinicians as a matter solely involving technological resources. We must remember clinical content's critical role in making technology useful for clinicians. A range of services exists along the continuum of service intensity in a typical community-based mental health entity, from outpatient to inpatient or residential services. Such complex organizations also serve multiple populations: children, adults, and the elderly. They may also serve multiple disability populations, such as substance abusers and the developmentally disabled. It is likely that each of these service levels and populations requires specialized clinical content. The development and implementation of such content is not a trivial exercise, especially since each of these content bundles has to be localized and tailored, to some extent, for the specific enterprise.

Thus, the full evolution of a pervasive computing environment, with its high degree of simultaneous access by multiple clinicians and the ready sharing of clinical information, depends on a full network infrastructure and implementation of multiple clinical content sets. Remember the fax machines: the full value of healthcare informatics only becomes evident when all nodes are fully networked. Viewed another way, the implementation of healthcare informatics is a long, incremental process, with a delayed value proposition. While individual clinicians will enjoy the benefits of such technology by an increase in their personal productivity, the full benefits to the clinical enterprise will be a trickle–flood phenomenon, with a long trickle cycle.

Another dimension to the development of network infrastructure, independent of clinical content, creates enormous value. One of the most striking aspects of the Internet is its ability to create and foster communities. Communities deal with interactive communication, and the Web is rich with interactive media. E-mail has been reason enough for people to purchase Web-based technology. The near viral spread of instant messaging (IM) reflects a desire for even more intense interfacing, telescoped in time and exquisitely targeted.

Wiring an enterprise regardless of size creates the likelihood that a wide variety of communities will be formed within it, including one that includes the parent enterprise itself. Clinicians will use this neural network to assist them in their duties, even though doing so increases their liability as well as their employer's, since e-mail and IM posts can be revealed to outsiders. A policy and procedural etiquette will develop over time that limits such liability. It is possible that legal case law will find creative ways to treat such communication, so that some protection is afforded this informal, open communication channel. If neither occurs, then inventive technologists will provide automatic deletion and "scrubbing" services that maintain this channel and limit liability. It is simply inconceivable that such community-building and communication-sparking capabilities will be killed off by the threat of increased liability.

As the threat of liability is channeled or constrained, by either technological or procedural means, the selfsame technologists will use this neural network to act as a systemwide "to-do list" service, automatically triggering reminders, prompts, and electronic nags of all types. However intrusive such a stream of reminders might be, clinicians clearly wish to shift the responsibility of recording everything on the carbon-based software inside their skulls to virtual memory prosthetics that reside on the network.

A final word about communities: there is no reason that communities must exclude the clients and consumers of behavioral health care. A commitment to pervasive computing means that the boundary between the enterprise and its consumers becomes more permeable. If all clinical content is on the network, then clients could conceivably have some level of access to it. Clinicians will not be the only ones with "casual accessibility" to network appliances. Clients could facilitate intake and assessments by filling out significant amounts of information prior to arriving at the physical service site. If intake and assessments could be managed, why not a sample treatment plan, guided by the same software used by the clinician? The point is to not replace the clinician, but to make the client–clinician interaction more collaborative. It should channel clinical time into higher value discussions related to client choices. This is not utopian rhetoric. Instead, it is a prediction that both clinicians and clients will arrive independently at such uses of this technology. This also includes the significantly impaired contingent, since diminished capacity does not equate to ignorance. Truly intuitive software should be obvious enough for use by a wide range of clients. For the instances where it is not, creative developers can make the necessary alterations.

The Analysis of Clinical Information: The Rise of Reflective Practice

The melding of clinical and technology transactions will create significant data warehouses, if we assume there will be pervasive computing development and an increased implementation of healthcare informatics. While these electronic storehouses will enable researchers to "slice and dice" the data in a myriad of ways, the real issue is whether this new ability will make any difference at the intervention practice level.

In the absence of feedback, there is no internal reflection. Intervention practice will be impacted only if the information from these storehouses is looped back to the clinician. Intervention plans and practice can be filtered through best-practice protocols and an ongoing stream of messages can be provided to the clinician, since information is quickly shared in a pervasive computing environment. This clinical "Big Brotherism" can be lessened substantially by making the access to such information optional. Younger, less experienced clinicians could be required or encouraged to use such clinical assistance during a probationary period, while the more seasoned utilize it only when desired.

All clinicians could access information about client treatment outcomes specific to their needs. Such information could be located on the clinician's personal clinical information portal, or "dashboard," and present automatically as part of a standard clinical profile on each client.

We have implicitly defined "reporting practice" as how the clinician enters clinical information into a pervasive computing environment. Reporting practice should also encompass how that environment or the system automatically presents client-specific information to the clinician. Automatic presentation can come from multiple data sources—the local enterprise system or multiple external systems. For example, the local system can present a listing of risk potentials for the client, as reported in the intake process; a listing of medications currently prescribed and any incidence of adverse reactions to them; and lab results. From the external systems, the clinician could view predicted milestones of accomplishment for comparable clients receiving similar interventions, the modal number of visits for clients with similar diagnoses, and so on. Such population-based information enables the clinician to weigh the effects of her interventions and trigger an important interior dialogue that could affect the amount and type of future interventions. Thus, the pervasive network is a two-way highway; the comparative data that it presents to the clinician create the capacity for reflection.

Conclusion

Narrowing the gap between clinical and technology transactions will require the integration of a broad range of technologies. While current pervasive computing technology is too primitive, costly, and incomplete for widespread use, it is worth noting that the Web has a short and limited history. What is expensive, highly customized, "roll-your-own technology" today will be an off-the-shelf commodity two years from now. Both the clinicians and their vendors must assume this progression and begin creating the clinical content necessary to make such technology useful. Clinicians and clients will test the limits of its possibilities only when the technology and content are in place, as they create new communities of interaction.

Bibliography

Balch DC, Warner DJ. Medical knowledge on demand—highlights from the third. *MD Comput* 1999;16(2):48–49.

Collen MF. The evolution of computer communications. *MD Comput* 2000;17(1):72.

Collen MF. Evolution of the user/computer interface: part 2, data output. *MD Comput* 2000;17(1):72.

Johnshoy-Currie CJ. Challenges in cyberpsych—the conference on behavioral informatics. *MD Comput* 1999;16(3):50–53.

Kiel JM, Cherry JC. Positive outcomes, lower costs: using net-based IT to manage care. *MD Comput* 2000;17(2):27–28.

McKenzie NC, Marks IM. Overcoming interface problems in computerized monitoring of clinical outcomes. *MD Comput* 1997;14(5):377–381.

Okstein CJ. XML: a key technology for sharing clinical information. *MD Comput* 1999;16(5):31.

Patel VL, Kaufman DR. Medical informatics and the science of cognition. *JAMIA* 1998;5(6):493–502.

Rees SE. Artificial intelligence and medical decision-making: exploring challenges and opportunities. *MD Comput* 1999;16(5):17.

Spath P. Case management—making the case for information systems. *MD Comput* 2000;17(3):40–44.

Tang PC, LaRosa MP, Newcomb C, Gorden S. Measuring the effects of reminders for outpatient influenza immunizations at the point of clinical opportunity. *JAMIA* 1999; 6(2):115–121.

Teich JM, Wrinn MM. Clinical decision support systems come of age. *MD Comput* 2000; 17(1):43.

Zafar A, Overhage MJ, McDonald CJ. Continuous speech recognition for clinicians. *JAMIA* 1999;6(3):195–204.

9
Improving Quality and Accountability Through Information Systems

CHARLES RUETSCH, DAVID M. WADELL, AND NAAKESH A. DEWAN

Quality improvement within health care is conceptually linked to patient outcomes. Though outcomes cannot often be directly measured, the goal of quality improvement is to improve patient outcomes in response to treatment. Payers of health insurance are increasingly focused on investment return, seeking maximal improvement in treatment outcomes for minimal premium dollars. Managed care companies are facing increasing scrutiny, and are being mandated to improve patient outcomes while continuing to contain costs.

Improvement in specific patient outcomes requires enhancements to specific care management and administrative processes within managed care companies. Increasing service availability, access, and care coordination have been the hallmarks of quality improvement in behavioral health care during the past decade. The gains in conservation of limited behavioral health benefits and in access to behavioral health providers have been marked. However, the types of data and data analyses outlined in this chapter suggest that outcomes within behavioral health care can be used to allow for a more targeted strategy for enhancing processes that make a difference in targeted patient populations. For example, recent studies show that quality improvement and outcomes data can be used to enable the most severely mentally ill populations, increasing the amount of time that they spend in community settings and of reducing the amount of time spent in hospital settings. Increased differentiation of response to treatment can be guided by quality improvement and outcomes data through the conduit of informatics.

Data are needed to guide the development of information systems that support the targeted enhancements in outcomes. Therefore, the quality of behavioral healthcare improvements is dependent on the availability of accurate, reliable data. Systematic evaluation of care management and delivery will require sophisticated information systems that can integrate data from multiple sources (clinical treatment records, clinical authorization information systems, claims payment systems, customer satisfaction and outcomes management systems, pharmacy records, and provider and facility databases). However, one must understand the history and application of quality improvement principles to behavioral health care before one can truly appreciate the information system requirements of today's delivery systems.

The focus of this chapter is on the real-life experiences and challenges of managed behavioral healthcare companies, most notably in their effort to measure and improve patient outcomes while containing both administrative and direct care costs. The informatics community has placed emphasis on the informatics solutions and challenges to develop and deploy solutions where currently none exist or where those that exist are not integrated. The chapter begins with a review of quality improvement in health care, followed by a brief review of outcomes and their role in quality improvement. The chapter then discusses the important role of informatics in quality improvement for managed behavioral health care as well as its challenges and future direction.

History of Quality in Health Care

The history of quality in health care can be traced to the mid-19th century. Florence Nightingale observed the lack of information in hospital records and deduced that to be the reason why some patients responded well to their treatments, while others seemed not to improve or to deteriorate. Several years passed before her observations could translate into action. In 1913, the American College of Surgeons was formed by a group of American physicians who were interested in understanding the variability of patient outcomes. This group published the first set of quality standards for hospitals. These early standards were centered on the development and use of clinical records to assess performance and explain variation. The college developed the Hospital Standardization Program, which measured hospital compliance with its standards, in 1917. This became the first systematic quality assurance process in health care, and it relied heavily on retrospective audits of patient charts and hospital policies.

The development and refinement of quality assurance standards continued, and others began to develop theoretical models to explain quality measurement. One of these was a model that described the relationship among structural elements, such as facility characteristics, technology/instrumentation available to the clinician, staff competence (education level, for example), and process elements like methods of diagnosis and treatment.[1] Donabedian's[1] model suggested that the two elements of structure and process accounted for the variation in outcomes observed across populations.

In the 1950s, the Joint Commission on Accreditation of Hospitals (JCAH) was formed to further the development of quality standards for healthcare delivery. An accreditation program was established whereby hospitals could voluntarily be measured against established standards through on-site surveys. Surveyors evaluated the hospitals' structure and processes through interviews and documentation reviews. These results were then used as proxies for quality of patient care measures; conclusions were drawn about the outcomes of care based on the evaluation of structure and process. Over time, the Joint Commission changed its name to the Joint Commission on Accreditation of Healthcare Organizations

(JCAHO) and expanded the standards to include other care settings and methods of treatment management.

The rapid rise of healthcare costs and fragmentation in the healthcare delivery system in the 1970s and 1980s led to the development of alternative healthcare delivery models, such as managed care. The management of care was through contracted networks of clinicians and facilities and required different measurement standards from those used in facility-based care. To assess and report on the quality of these new managed health plans, an independent, not-for-profit organization called the National Committee for Quality Assurance (NCQA) was formed. Like JCAHO, the NCQA developed quality standards and established an accreditation program, which was offered voluntarily to these new managed care organizations as a way of demonstrating to the public that they provided quality services. Following in the footsteps of previously established accreditation organizations, the NCQA diversified by developing certification and accreditation programs for related healthcare organizations. In 1995, the NCQA began developing standards for evaluating managed behavioral healthcare organizations (MBHOs). These standards, in addition to a related accreditation program, were completed and implemented in 1997. In response, the MBHOs developed quality assurance departments that focused on measuring and modifying programs to ensure compliance with the NCQA's standards for the MBHO.

Continuous Quality Improvement

American industry embraced a new quality philosophy during the 1980s and 1990s: Total Quality Management (TQM) or Continuous Quality Improvement (CQI). The theories behind TQM are based on the works of Walter Shewhart, W. Edwards Deming, Joseph M. Juran, and Philip Crosby. Walter Shewhart,[2] while working as a physicist at Bell Laboratories in the 1920s, developed both statistical techniques to help measure process variability and a method to reduce variation to acceptable levels. This method has come to be known as the "Plan, Do, Check, Act" method of quality improvement:

Plan—identify opportunity for improvement
Do—implement interventions
Check—measure affect of interventions
Act—adjust interventions/change interventions.

Deming[3] used Shewhart's techniques and an understanding of organizational culture to launch the Japanese quality revolution in the 1950s. He taught the Japanese to utilize Shewhart's model as a continuous cycle of Plan, Do, Check, and Act until the product variation remained within an acceptable range. Juran[4] began lecturing in Japan during the mid-1950s on management theory, strategic planning, and quality management. He built on the statistical and cultural foundation established by Deming to focus on the elimination of waste and redoing.

Philip Crosby[5] presented a well-defined quality management program for creating awareness and changing attitudes within an organization, especially toward establishing and maintaining quality products and services. This program was based on the idea that quality is the responsibility of every worker and that it reflects the attitudes of management. As a result, leadership in quality improvement must be provided by top management. While this philosophy began in the manufacturing industry, it was not long before other employers began incorporating these theories into their own work settings.

Healthcare Quality Assurance Evolves into Quality Improvement

By the mid-1980s, visionaries in healthcare quality began to explore the application of TQM principles to health care. Donald Berwick[6] used the analogy of "identifying and eliminating bad apples" to explain the *quality assurance* model of inspection and outliers removal that was, at that time, typical in most healthcare settings. He proposed a *systems-based* model, which was based on statistically analyzing the results of patient care and supporting administrative functions to determine the cause of patient variation. Variation in patient outcomes was analyzed, and then root causes were systematically addressed and, when possible, eliminated. Berwick's model clearly shared many of the principles of CQI, and *quality improvement* within health care was born.

The accreditation organizations followed Berwick's lead. JCAHO modified its standards to reflect measures of an organization's leadership, cultural foundation, planning, and use of continuous quality improvement methods in what they called the "Agenda for Change." Likewise, NCQA also underwent standard revisions. They reassessed how to evaluate managed care organizations on their ability to identify opportunities for improvement, analyze data to determine the leading barriers to improvement, implement appropriate interventions, and measure results. NCQA established this process as a set of standards for quality improvement and called them quality improvement activities (QIAs). QIAs became, and remain, the preferred method of managed care organizations for demonstrating successful CQI implementation of improved quality of care and service. Dewan and Carpenter[7] reviewed the performance measurement and quality improvement efforts in behavioral health care.

Quality Improvement in Behavioral Health Care

The evolution of quality improvement in behavioral health care began with the incorporation of principles implemented in general medicine. In the past, behavioral healthcare organizations attempted to apply the established quality assurance standards for medical care to their own treatment and delivery models. Greater attention has recently been focused on the development of quality improvement principles specifically for the management and delivery of behavioral healthcare. Though national accreditation agencies such as NCQA and American Accreditation Healthcare Commission (aka URAC) employ many of the same standards for evaluating the effectiveness of MBHOs and managed care organizations (MCOs), the skills that are required to prepare for accreditation surveys as well as participate on the survey teams are quite different. Though a full discussion of this topic is beyond the scope of this chapter, it is clear that the types of data used for behavioral healthcare quality improvement and outcomes studies are quite different from those used to address similar issues within general medicine. Though quality improvement activities have been part of both the MBHO and MCO standards, the processes that are improved and the outcomes that are measured are quite different.

A case study of a quality improvement philosophy implemented at an MBHO is Magellan Behavioral Health. Magellan Health Services[8] is the United States' largest and most comprehensive specialty behavioral health managed care organization, with responsibility for the care management of approximately 70 million individuals nationwide (*www.Magellanhealth.com*). Magellan takes the historical perspectives and blends them into four broad concepts that are used to support the CQI program:

1. *Customer driven:* Magellan acknowledges its multiple sources of influence, loosely grouped as customer constituencies including members, patients, families, payers (e.g., health plans, employers, state/municipal government), providers, facilities, regulatory agencies, and accreditation bodies. Each of these customers has specific expectations with regard to its relationship to Magellan, and these expectations are translated into measurable performance standards. Magellan's concept of quality is achieved through meeting customer expectations, then continuing to improve to reach the goal of excellence.
2. *Focused on systemic issues rather than individuals:* Magellan recognizes the fact that all performed activities within the organization are processes. Each process is a sequence of steps that, when combined, result in some measurable outcome. Processes within each functional area are linked together and ultimately result in the products or services that are delivered to the customers. No process is perfect; flaws in this instance are called "barriers to excellence." Barriers are parts of a process that prohibit the system from reaching its potential or highest possible performance level. They are often integral to how employees complete job tasks, including the way they communicate with others and record central events (e.g., clinical information during an intake call). Barriers are not people; they are not underperforming staff, nor are they patients who are noncompliant with treatment regimens. Within a system such as an MBHO, examples of barriers include lack of effective coordination of providers, treatment facilities, community resources, and transportation, all of which may be needed at points during the recovery of a person after a mental health hospitalization. As a result, Magellan focuses its quality improvement efforts on removing barriers within its many processes, rather than focusing on individual outliers.

   For example, barriers within the care management system that may impact telephone performance (such as the average answering speed) can include staff schedules (adequacy during peak times), types of incoming calls (care management calls, complaints, claims calls), and talk time. To identify barriers, outcomes and process data are needed. Systems that track cases through the authorization for care process, that quickly route high priority calls to licensed clinicians, and that effectively capture and report clinician competence all need further development to better support the quality improvement (QI) process. Further, through aggregation, trends and patterns in performance can be identified and barriers eventually removed from systems that affect large populations.

3. *Employee involvement and empowerment:* Magellan embraces a culture of line-level staff involvement and empowerment. This is consistent with their belief that line staff are the ones most familiar with customer expectations and the processes they follow each day. Magellan achieves an integration of quality improvement within operations by involving and empowering employees throughout all steps of the QI process. This integration allows each employee equal responsibility for the quality of services delivered to customers.

4. *Outcomes-based decision making:* Magellan uses data for a number of processes, including identifying processes that have strong effects on outcomes, identifying opportunities for improvement, evaluating barriers to determine appropriate interventions and the outcomes of key processes, determining whether or not interventions are effective in improving member care and service, and measuring the extent to which it meets or exceeds customer expectations. Data are preferred over anecdotal statements, since they provide objective facts about operational performance, minimize subjectivity, and can be trended over time and across multiple systems of care delivery. Furthermore, data can be measured more specifically over time, thus providing a mechanism for tracking improvement. Magellan Behavioral Health has adopted or developed 26 measures of performance that are linked to member care or service. They include clinical indicators such as readmission to acute inpatient care, attendance at aftercare, and provider compliance with accepted clinical practice guidelines. Also included are core service indicators such as the speed with which member calls are answered and the speed with which member complaints or appeals are resolved. These indicators are measured using the same methodology across all regional offices and represent one of the largest databases of care and service performance in the MBHO industry. These data can be trended not only over time but also between regions, populations, benefit structures, and internationally. The sources of these data are computer systems that capture and store data and transform them into information needed to support quality improvement initiatives.

Quality Improvement Activities: An Application of CQI

Magellan's model for implementing its CQI philosophy is the quality improvement activity (QIA). QIAs are ideal for documenting operational improvements in care and services, and are mechanisms that help structure the task of improving complex processes. The most successful QIAs combine CQI tools: research methods, sound outcomes-based decision support, and expert knowledge in the content area being improved. When CQI principles and methodology are implemented well, and evidence is collected as part of everyday operations, the QIA report compilation is a description of the process and evidence of improvement.

CQI Cycle

Magellan's CQI model is closely aligned with NCQA's QIA process and relies on the identification and elimination of barriers to excellence; this process consequently fosters improvement in performance. Performing CQI on a process, such as care or network management, is a complex endeavor. Therefore, Magellan's model for QIA development presents the improvement process as a series of small steps:

• Identification of opportunities for improvement
• Analysis of barriers
• Development of interventions
• Implementation of interventions
• Tracking performance improvement

These steps are part of an ongoing improvement cycle (Fig. 9.1). The cycle begins with systematic performance measurement and opportunity for improvement identification (performance areas that could be improved). Once opportunities for improvement are identified, they are prioritized based on criteria such as relevance to member well-being and feasibility of change. Once the highest priority opportunities have been chosen, barriers to improvement are identified and interventions are developed and implemented to remove their effect on performance. Improvements in member care and services are monitored through re-

QIA Cycle

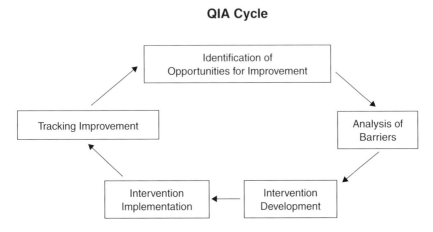

FIGURE 9.1 Quality improvement cycle in a managed behavioral health organization.

measurement of performance and comparison of remeasurement to baseline performance. If greater improvement is desired after one cycle, the QIA cycle may be repeated. Otherwise, improvement resources may be refocused on other highly prioritized opportunities for improvement.

Improvement in Existing Programs

CQI, by definition, provides structure to help improve existing processes. Within Magellan, the CQI process is applied to bring about programmatic changes, including the following:

1. Enhancing aftercare coordination
2. Enhancing management of high risk or fragile patients
3. Increasing compliance with preventive health screening through methods such as reminders and incentives
4. Improving the thoroughness of screening for comorbid substance abuse among depressed patients
5. Improving access to treatment.

However, CQI methods can be applied toward the improvement of any process and seeking care management input helps staff identify the highest priority activities.

Outcomes and Systemic Health Management Issues

Managed care is a system that was developed to manage a population's health benefits. The system is a confluence of policies, procedures, practices, information, and various information technologies that are used together to support care management decisions. This section focuses on the use of outcomes information in the ongoing design of managed care models. This means that outcomes can be used to identify opportunities to improve policies, procedures, practices, and technology that are used to care for the behavioral health of any population. Three applications within a large MBHO are presented, along with a brief discussion of how informatics affects these issues and makes resolution feasible where it was not possible even five years ago.

Aftercare Coordination

In 1992, nearly 40 million people in the United States experienced some type of mental disorder.[9] Lifetime estimates of mental illness prevalence are even higher,[10] thus making it comparable to that of many physical illnesses.[11] Although suicide remains one of the most serious consequences of mental illness, other social and economic consequences underscore the need for aggressive prevention and treatment efforts.[9]

It is important to continue treatment after discharging patients from an inpatient facility. Without continuity of services, many patients discontinue taking their medication and relapse into symptomatic behavior.[12] Ongoing services in a less restrictive environment prevent the occurrence of many adverse effects and help to assure that gains made during hospitalization are not lost. Outpatient visits within 30 days of discharge allow behavioral healthcare practitioners to detect early posthospitalization reactions and medication problems. Furthermore, follow-up services reduce the rate of readmission to hospital programs.[11,13]

Exactly how to increase the number of patients who attend and continue to attend aftercare following discharge from acute care is less clear than the potential impact of aftercare attendance on member well-being. Many questions remain unanswered:

• How does outreach affect attendance?
• Are some patients more ready to engage in aftercare than others?[14,15]
• What are the differential effects of various approaches to aftercare coordination?
• Is there value in matching patients with different approaches to aftercare based on patient characteristics such as social support, motivation, diagnosis, previous treatment history, or medical comorbidity?

Focused studies that address specific changes to the process of aftercare coordination, as well as their effect on aftercare attendance and subsequent re-hospitalization needs, will shed some light on these issues. Performance indicators, such as the percent of recently discharged patients who attend at least one aftercare appointment within 7 days, and the percent readmitted to acute inpatient care within 30 days, are quite helpful. However, to see measurable improvements in the well-being of the MBHO's membership, greater detail is needed in the form of more data from three sources: patients, providers, and care management staff.

Patient information within managed care administrative data systems typically includes basic information such as age, gender, and race. Though the enrollment process requests other demographic information from members, it is usually optional and left blank, thus resulting in data that are not representative of the population. To better understand the population, many managed care companies are conducting membership surveys, particularly of the treated population. Random samples from these surveys answer questions about members' social support system, medical problems, substance abuse problems, and other patient descriptors that help MBHOs understand how to improve existing programs. The resulting data can then be used to help improve existing programs and plan new programs. In the example that addresses aftercare coordination, patient information may be used to determine whether diagnosis, severity of illness, or treatment history are related to a patient's attendance at aftercare with only simple reminders, or whether patients with longer treatment histories require ongoing reminders and coordination after attending the first session to ensure continuation with a treatment regimen.

Provider and care manager profile data are typically more easily acquired than are data for members. Provider information is essential to the credentialing process. The desire to be accepted into an MBHO's provider network motivates providers to make specific information available to MBHO staff. Information such as the provider's training, degree, background, and specialty are part of the credentialing process. Likewise, care managers are often hired in part based on their training, degree, experience, and specialty. Added to this information are their supervisor's observations of specific skills and reviews of their patient charts. These data provide a rich platform of information from which may be developed care management decision support systems.

However, changes in programs must go beyond focused studies, and findings must be incorporated into operations. These applications require information technology that delivers the patient profile, provider profile, and recommendations for aftercare coordination procedures to thousands of care managers who speak with patients and providers on a daily basis about their aftercare plans and compliance. These systems must be easy to navigate and capable of providing information from several disparate databases simultaneously. Additionally, they must provide information in real time, instantaneously.

Provider Performance

Equally important to coordinating care is maintaining a highly effective provider network. Traditionally, provider performance has been monitored through audits of hospitals and provider offices, such as those by the Commission on Accreditation of Rehabilitation Services (CARF) and by JCAHO. In addition to site visits, a number of patient charts typically are reviewed for adherence to clinical standards and expected levels of documentation. Within the past five years, JCAHO and other accreditation agencies have begun to focus on patient-treatment outcomes (e.g., ORYX®). The rationale is that patient-treatment outcomes are the single best indicator of quality of patient care. All else held constant, higher quality providers are those whose patients get better faster, stay better longer, and have fewer complaints and adverse incidents. Currently, medical outcomes measurement is in many ways better established than its behavioral health counterpart. Therefore, behavioral health still relies heavily on measuring provider process, documentation standards, and compliance with clinical practice guidelines as proxies for outcomes and provider performance.

Provider audits typically generate tremendous amounts of paper. Checklists, patient chart excerpts, and utilization statistics need to be available for auditors to complete a thorough audit. Web-based applications are beginning to be developed, and audits of both MBHO and provider offices can be completed in their entirety using these applications. They have the advantage of being interactive with the user, who is entering information into the Web database as well as being prompted to locate and record specific information. In addition, these applications make available to the auditors information from provider and member databases within the MBHO. For example, auditors at a provider office may look up the provider's average number of sessions, readmission rate, patient-treatment outcomes (when they are available), satisfaction, and complaints—all while conducting the audit. As with any centralized system, Web-based applications make training and changes in protocol easier. The application needs to be updated only once and the protocol is updated for all auditors. Further, the quality of the auditor's work can be monitored for compliance with protocols. Patterns of audit findings can be analyzed to reveal auditors who tend to focus on certain weaknesses while failing to address others. Opportunities for auditor training can be identified easily, and training materials can be developed to address specific needs. Continued monitoring of auditors' results will reveal the level of success of the training, as well as other opportunities for improvement.

Access to Services

Several barriers to access exist within managed care. Provider density compared to membership density and need for services, access within time standards, and delay time awaiting authorization for reimbursement are all barriers that slow the patient's access to needed care. Assessing the competence of providers and maintaining a high-quality network was in small part addressed in the previous section. This section focuses on barriers within the authorization process.

Within most MBHOs over the past 10 years, when a patient requires services, either the patient/advocate or the provider contacts the MBHO and requests authorization for service (reimbursement). The MBHO representative then verifies the patient's eligibility for benefits and the need for services. The result is either an authorization, which means that the provider can render services with a guarantee of reimbursement from the MBHO, or a nonauthorization, which means that services cannot be reimbursed. Any delay in the authorization decision process has the potential to delay the beginning of treatment. Possible points of delay include provider availability to contact the MBHO and telephone hold time.

Web-based applications have been developed to increase the efficiency of provider inquiries regarding member enrollment information. For example, within some benefit structures, authorization of outpatient care is not necessary for reimbursement. However, providers still must confirm member eligibility and guard against members' misrepresenting their insurance status or level of benefit exhaustion. Currently, providers can log onto the Web sites of some MBHOs and, through a series of passwords and other security systems, access member eligibility information. These systems are interactive in that once eligibility is verified, the provider can log a request for reimbursement after the session is completed and a claim submitted. This application saves the providers time in that they no longer need to contact the MBHO via telephone to verify eligibility and seek authorization for reimbursement for routine care.

Behavioral Health Informatics for Quality Improvement

Consistent with this environment, behavioral healthcare informatics initially focused on the fundamental necessities of doing business: authorization and claims processing. These initial systems were generally written in PIC or COBOL programming languages, were relatively inflexible with regard to configuration and extensibility, and required expensive programming resources for generating canned reports. These systems were commonly implementations of existing managed healthcare applications, and were configured to support only those procedure codes and diagnostic categories associated with the delivery of behavioral health specialty services. These systems operated as single-tier information systems, with users connecting either via dial-up or direct connection via dumb terminals (or terminal emulators running on desktop PCs).

During the early 1990s, the information requirements to support quality management and accreditation requirements rapidly outgrew the capabilities of existing behavioral health information system infrastructures (this problem was not distinct to the behavioral healthcare sector; it was, and continues to be, a significant challenge for the healthcare industry as a whole). At the same time, the demand for reliable data regarding quality of member care and services far outpaced the availability of affordable mechanisms to replace or supplement existing data sources.

Consequently, a grass roots effort began in many managed behavioral health organizations to harness the skills of employees who had a basic understanding of database structure and expertise in inexpensive database management tools. Realizing the opportunity represented by having an electronic record of customer contacts with automated data collection integrated seamlessly into the work flow of general operations, industry leaders began to take notice of these "home-grown" information systems and evaluate them for implementation on a more global scale.

Using some of the more sophisticated grass roots projects as a springboard, several managed behavioral health organizations hired programmers and established project teams to develop scalable applications to support the growing business requirement for elaborate data acquisition, reporting, and analysis. These visionary companies realized that the ability to demonstrate an active program for improving quality and healthcare outcomes would become a competitive advantage in the short term, and a "ticket for entry" in the long term for continued success as a healthcare company. The early adopters could become market leaders and set the minimum standard for new entrants to the marketplace.

The first generation of applications to support business operations and data requirements are typically based on two-tier integrated technology, with the front-end application containing the business logic and the second tier composed of a scalable enterprise database management system (DBMS). The applications are generally written in very flexible, third-generation programming languages and are commonly developed as a stand-alone systems, distinct from the legacy authorization and claims systems. Among the advantages of these systems are the following:

- Intuitive, user friendly graphical user interface (GUI)
- Reduced paper documentation
- Increased contemporaneous availability of data/documentation across distinct users

• Significant improvement in work-flow efficiency
• A reduction in manual data collection mechanisms and improved reliability of data.

Though advances in system design currently allow for flexible integration of intuitive user interfaces with powerful database engines, source data typically require duplication from legacy authorization and claims payment systems. Therefore, many challenges to data availability and integrity inherent within the older legacy systems continued to influence the effectiveness of the newer, more sophisticated systems.

Data Source Challenges

The benefit of sophisticated information systems to support quality and outcomes initiatives is dependent on the usefulness of the data elements captured in those systems. Unfortunately, in behavioral care, many data source challenges exist that can inhibit the effective use of this information.

Measurement

A population's behavioral health is difficult to measure. There are rarely external or biological markers to most mental illnesses. As a result, the most widely used methods for assessing mental health are patient self-report and provider observation. Both methods are costly to implement and have historically required a great deal of manual labor for collecting and managing the data. Population-based studies often take years to mature and result in data that are of little use to an industry that changes as quickly as does behavioral health. Behavioral health household surveys, census information, and other large survey and polling efforts provide some information, but are costly and often not focused enough to identify specific problems in care management systems. For example, many household surveys capture information such as the incidence and initiation of substance abuse among teens; however, they do not typically collect information about the effect of new managed care programs on substance abuse (teen outreach, drug awareness, and prevention). In contrast, highly detailed and in-depth information is available from individuals who access care through a managed care system. These individuals can also be the most informative group identifying effectiveness of current managed care models and potential for improvements.

Another significant measurement challenge is confidentiality. Individuals by nature are reluctant to provide accurate information about their demographics or health status if it can be traced back to their identities. Legitimate fears regarding the release of such information have prompted federal and state regulations limiting the ability to collect and use information that is vital to demonstrate the effectiveness of treatment or the efficiency of administrative services. Consider a simple study to determine the cost/benefit of three treatment options for major depression: (1) individual therapy alone, (2) individual therapy combined with drug therapy, and (3) drug therapy alone. In today's complicated healthcare system, such a study might require data from multiple sources, including a behavioral healthcare vendor, a general medical HMO, a third-party claims administrator, a pharmacy benefits manager, and others. Each of these entities can be prevented from sharing the data required to conduct such a study by their own confidentiality policies, by customers' expectations, by state or federal regulations, and by accreditation standards.

Lack of Data Standards and Definitions

In addition to the confidentiality issues entailed in collecting and combining data, the physical ability of organizations to link data from varying sources can be a challenge. For example, a customer complaint database may track complaints from providers by provider number, while the claims department tracks payment to providers by tax ID number. If there is not a common data element, it would be difficult if not impossible to pinpoint provider-related potential causes for complaints about timely claims payments. Further, the plethora of mergers and acquisitions of the 1980s and 1990s left many behavioral healthcare companies with multiple information systems. These information systems superficially appear to collect the same data. However, analysis of detailed data definitions often reveals that these systems are collecting vastly different information. In one system, a confirmed appointment is identified only after a follow-up call is made to a provider's office; in another system, that confirmed appointment is recorded when patients indicate that they intend to follow through. Though these two indicators are both called "attendance at aftercare," they clearly measure different outcomes. Therefore, combining this information for quality purposes could have deleterious effects on the quality improvement initiative.

Communication

Another significant challenge is communication between the quality improvement staff and the information system programmers. This vital communication link can be akin to attempted communication between two individuals who speak different languages. A common scenario begins with a request by the QI staff for programming or report generation to support a specific improvement opportunity. The information systems professional listens intently to the request, but often does not understand its purpose. Nonetheless, the information systems professional writes the program codes necessary to accomplish the task and sends these codes back to the QI staff for approval prior to initiating the work. The QI staff reviews the document, which, because of the programming language, is unintelligible, and approves the document because, "they are information systems professionals and they must know what they are doing." After hours of programming and report generation, the final product does not result in the information required by the QI staff. This lack of effective communication often inhibits the effective and efficient quality improvement outcome initiative.

While data source challenges such as these can have a serious impact on quality and outcomes initiatives, mechanisms exist to reduce their effect. Organizations must embrace a common standard for confidentiality. More effective communication with patients about the value of specific shared data can be combined with appropriate release of information forms that allow for the sharing of data between caregivers and payers; this will reduce the liability associated with these system quality improvement and outcomes projects. These forms can be supported by interdisciplinary, interorganizational review boards whose responsibilities include the review of methodologies to ensure appropriate confidentiality of information. Likewise, solid planning around data definitions and elements prior to building new information systems will ensure their connectivity to existing systems. The construction of data warehouses to assimilate data from different sources with different definitions can also be helpful to organizations faced with multiple systems. These data warehouses can be constructed to include transformations, where possible, to align the definitions of disparate data sources.

Finally, training and using business analysts to interface between information systems programmers and quality improvement staff can alleviate communication issues. Business analysts are highly trained individuals who are knowledgeable about the data elements and definitions within the information system and have a solid understanding of the behavioral healthcare industry. These individuals often write the initial specifications for programming needs based on discussion with the QI staff, and approve the programming documents through discussion with the information systems programmer. In conclusion, data source challenges can be minimized by understanding their impact and developing proactive solutions to address them.

Data Interface

The lack of interface between the clinical/service/quality management information system and the legacy authorization and claims systems left significant opportunities for improving work flow efficiency and data sharing in the next generation of applications (users were still required to use the clinical/service/quality management information system in parallel with the authorization and claims systems).

In response to these challenges, applications were developed specifically to integrate user-friendly interfaces with legacy systems (most notably authorization and claims systems) and continued feature evolution to support a rapidly changing business environment. During this phase of evolution, programmers created asynchronous, bidirectional data conversion procedures between the clinical/service/quality management information system and the authorization and claims systems. Additionally, these data conversion interfaces were used to expand the capabilities of the clinical/service/quality management information system to incorporate updates from member eligibility and provider databases. Now, the care managers or customer service representatives of the managed behavioral health organization would have the majority of information required to perform their primary job duties (member eligibility, documentation of previous contacts, provider network participation) from a single user interface. Additionally, authorizations could be issued in the clinical/service/quality management information system, eliminating the necessity to work in parallel systems.

Information for a Client-Centered Approach to Care Management: MBHO Illustrations

Information is the single most empowering element within a managed behavioral health program. Front-line staff who speak with patients, providers, and family members on a daily basis need information to adequately recommend and support a behavioral health treatment plan of action. More information is not always more empowering. However, when specific information needs are not met, care decisions may not result in the best possible patient outcomes. The middle ground between inadequate information and information overload is the focus of research on informatics within MBHOs. Effective informatics provides needed information in a timely fashion and in a format that is flexile enough to allow the end user to mine more detailed information when needed. What follows are examples of informatic applications that were developed to improve specific member care processes within an MBHO.

Clinical Information Systems and Aftercare Coordination

The clinical information system used by Magellan is used to query data that are essential to authorizing care. End-users have at their disposal member eligibility and benefit structure information; service utilization history and remaining benefits; and provider information including location, contact information, and specialty. Searches can be initiated by member ID, provider name or ID, dates of service, or authorization number. This information is evaluated in real time, usually during a request for services. The design and technology are not new, and most of these functions have been widely available on a variety of legacy mainframe systems. However, the architecture takes advantage of multiple tiered system development and integrates both old and new technologies as well as old and new data platforms. For example, member information is loaded into the system from eligibility tapes just as this had been done on legacy systems for the past decade. However, provider information, treatment history, and scheduled care management activities are either part of the clinical information system data files or are ported in from other external files either in real time or scheduled replication.

The Magellan clinical information system is more robust than most systems in that it provides user prompts for scheduled actions. For example, when a member is admitted to acute hospitalization, the system automatically prompts the care manager in charge of the case to initiate discussion with the hospital staff concerning discharge plans. As part of discharge planning, hospital staff members identify an aftercare provider and schedule an appointment that is captured in the system. On the day after the scheduled aftercare appointment, the same care manager is prompted to contact the aftercare provider to confirm that the member attended the appointment. In the case of a missed appointment, the system will provide the member's contact information to the care manager, who then attempts to contact the member, identify barriers to attendance at aftercare, arrange for help to overcome the barriers, and schedule another appointment. All of these activities are automated within a single user interface.

The Magellan Clinical Information System and UM (Utilization Management) Decision Agreement

Medical necessity criteria (MNC) are policies that state when and under what conditions member care will be reimbursed. Licensed clinicians conduct most of the assessments and determine the need for treatment based on the medical necessity criteria. The criteria are based on accepted standards of practice and guidelines for care. It is the agreement between the care manager's assessment of member need for treatment and the MNC that determines the level of care that will be authorized for reimbursement. The MNC are reviewed annually against industry and professional standards and updated in the clinical information system. A simple series of questions answered by a member or clinician are entered into a screen, and an algorithm then identifies what level of the MNC is satisfied. The result is a message indicating the level of reimbursement that is authorized.

   Both of the examples described in this section are driven by information that is "pushed out" to the care managers who are the end-users. The section that follows outlines the next generation of systems that will be based on assumptions concerning the health needs of a population. These systems will use outcomes, provider profile, and audit and utilization information to develop care management models for maintaining the highest level of behavioral health and population well being.

Smart and Self-Correcting Systems

Real-time knowledge of population treatment need and patient-treatment outcomes is crucial to continued development of effective care management models. One of the major challenges that faces MBHOs and behavioral health providers is balancing the need to provide effective care while keeping costs low. To manage cost and quality of care effectively, fiscal and quality processes must be combined in real time by those staff members who are making medical necessity decisions. However, care managers typically have not had the information technologies that combine these two data streams. QI staff and care managers have traditionally monitored treatment quality in solely clinical terms. Only now are they beginning to understand how to use fiscal and outcomes data in combination with MNC information to effectively manage the well-being of a covered population.

To address these needs, several companies have developed systems for collecting and managing patient-treatment outcomes data for group practices and MBHOs. Such systems include automated data capture and reporting. Case level reports include admission indication for treatment, historical psychiatric information, and progress in treatment. Aggregate reports include facility as well as level of admission severity and outcomes data. Some systems make case level reports available in nearly real time (less than an hour). However, few combine outcomes, epidemiological data (e.g., regional population need for treatment), utilization management, and fiscal data for care decision support. Missing from this and many other systems is an automated process for comparing service utilization and patient treatment outcomes. Such analyses are often relegated to special projects' departments of most MBHOs, and there has been little standardization of methods or benchmarking of outcomes.

Though each of the systems in this section illustrate the potential of integrating several otherwise disparate data sources, these systems rely largely on enterprise databases. Missing are links and ports to repositories external to the MBHO company.

Current trends toward improving the efficacy of care management within behavioral healthcare delivery systems are creating an impetus toward a level of health data integration never before seen in the industry. Managed healthcare organizations are now beginning to share quality improvement and outcomes information with other sectors of the healthcare continuum. Interfaces with pharmaceutical benefits companies, primary care physicians, and health plans provide the potential for sharing information and addressing problems such as cost-shifting, inefficient or duplicative service utilization and waste, and coordination of care across disciplines. These motives, combined with regulatory requirements for collaboration, are setting the stage for industry-shaping new paradigms for health information systems. The primary limitation of the existing information infrastructure for the healthcare industry as a whole is the focus on enterprise-specific solutions with little to no portability of data from one vendor to the next. However, technologies such as object-oriented programming and object-oriented database management systems (which easily scale for thousands of users and are capable of storing terabytes of data), extensible markup language (XML), distributed object technologies, wireless and hand-held technologies, highly secure virtual private networks (VPNs), and affordable high-speed Internet connectivity provide great potential solutions to current and emerging demands within the industry.

Conclusions and Recommendations

With treatment costs largely under control, the role of MBHOs is to improve the quality of member care and services within the current cost of care structures. Several government agencies and independent healthcare policy institutes have called for managed care systems to focus on improvement of clinical outcomes as evidence of success in increasing quality of care. Improving quality of care requires parallel increases in the effectiveness of the care management process. Effectiveness of care management is dependent on the specificity, validity, and timeliness of treatment and disease history of individual cases and comparable populations. Though these data are available as part of special projects, they are typically not available within the time constraints used for making care management decisions. These data must be available and presented in understandable bits to care management staff within minutes of request for care. Otherwise, members are left waiting for an informed care management decision, or care management decisions are made on inadequate information.

Information systems quickly identify needed information, across platforms, and calculate and present information to end-users within specific templates. However, the rate at which care management models are evolving within MBHOs requires a great deal of flexibility in addition to speed and accuracy. Such a system would need both the database query power of mainframe technology as well as customizability and flexibility of Web or local database technology. Further, the system would have to be both read and write from the local client to the local database and centralized data repository. Multiple data entry formats [e.g., IVR (Integrated Verbal Response), Web, scannable forms, keyboard] would all be needed as large MBHOs often service several regional offices and providers both with varying information technology capabilities. Larger MBHOs have the resources to build such systems themselves, while smaller companies will no doubt rely on external vendors and consultants. In either case, several technologies will be linked together, the information will be passed between them quickly, and the care of millions of people will depend on the accuracy, timeliness, and validity of the information that appears on a care manager and/or provider's computer screen. There is little time for error trapping and little tolerance for error.

Acknowledgments. The authors would like to thank Clarissa Marques, Joann Albright, Michael Kubica, and Gloria Uhl for their review and comments on previous versions of this chapter. We also thank Alisa Chestler, Erin Somers, and Pat Savory for their support and consultation during document preparation.

References

1. Donabedian A. *Explorations in Quality Assessment and Monitoring.* Ann Arbor, MI: Health Administration Press, 1980.
2. Shewhart W. *Economic Control of Quality of Manufactured Product.* New York: Van Nostrand, 1931.
3. Deming W. *Out of the Crisis.* Cambridge, MA: MIT Center for Advanced Engineering Study, 1986.
4. Juran JM. *Juran on Leadership for Quality: An Executive Handbook.* New York: The Free Press, 1989.

5. Crosby PB. *Quality Without Tears: The Art of Hassle-Free Management.* New York: McGraw-Hill, 1980.

6. Berwick DM. Continuous improvement as an ideal in healthcare. *N Engl J Med* 1989;320:53–56.

7. Dewan NA, Carpenter D. Performance measurement in healthcare delivery systems. *Psychol Biol Assess Turn Century* 1997;16:81–102.

8. Magellan Health Services. Transforming knowledge into results, 1998. *http://www. magellanhealth.com.*

9. National Center for Health Statistics. Health People 2000 Review, 1998–1999. Priority area 6. Mental Health and Mental Disorders. 1998:78–80.

10. Kessler RC, McGonagle KA, Zhao S. Lifetime and 12-month prevalence of DSM-IIIR psychiatric disorders in the U.S. *Arch Gen Psychiatry* 1994;51:8–19.

11. National Advisory Mental Health Council. Healthcare reform for Americans severe mental illness: report of the National Advisory on Mental Health Council. *Am J Psychiatry* 1993;150:1447–1464.

12. Daley D, Zuckoff A. Improving compliance with the initial outpatient session among discharged inpatient dual diagnosis clients. *Social Work,* 1998;43:470–473.

13. Schoenbaum SC, Cookson D, Stelovich S. Postdischarge follow-up of psychiatric inpatients and readmission in an HMO setting. *Psychiatric Serv* 1995;46:943–945.

14. Prochaska JO. *Systems of Psychotherapy: A Transtheoretical Analysis.* Homewood, IL: Dorsey, 1979.

15. Prochaska JO, DiClemente CC. Stages of change in the modification of problem behaviors. In: Hersen M, Eosler RM, Miller PM, eds. *Progress in Behavior Modification.* Sycamore, IL: Sycamore, 1992:184–214.

10
Decision Support 2000+: A New Information System for Public Mental Health Care

MARILYN J. HENDERSON, SARAH L. MINDEN, AND RONALD W. MANDERSCHEID

The federal government has been very involved in supporting the data standards and infrastructure development processes that are driving the e-healthcare boom today. Historically, the federal government has supported efforts to develop common data standards in the mental health arena through efforts at the Center for Mental Health Services within the Substance Abuse and Mental Health Services Administration and the National Institute of Mental Health within the Alcohol, Drug Abuse, and Mental Health Administration. This chapter provides insight into the government's efforts in the United States as we enter the new millennium. Current efforts, however, would not have been possible without the groundbreaking efforts of the 1970s and 1980s.

History of Data Standards Development

The federal government set up the Model Reporting Area for Mental Hospital Statistics to work on data standards for hospitals. With the shift from institution-based to community-based services, the Mental Health Statistics Improvement Program (MHSIP) was initiated in 1976, to expand the federal government's collaboration with states in developing and implementing data standards and information systems. Initial standards were prepared in 1983 that encompassed both hospital and community programs.[1] These standards were based on the mental health organization as the principal reporting unit.

MHSIP continued to change along with the mental health system, and in its 1989 report, *Data Standards for Mental Health Decision Support Systems* (the now famous FN 10),[2] MHSIP recommended standards and presented minimum data sets for patient/client, event, human resources, and financial and organizational data. Within FN 10, the clinical event was viewed as the basic unit of the system, to which patient/client, provider, and financial information could be linked within an organizational framework (Fig. 10.1).

The FN 10 data standards were voluntarily adopted by many state mental health authorities. They are still viewed as the codification of the recommended mini-

**1989 Mental Health Statistics
Improvement Program (MHSIP)**

◆━━━◆

Domains for Data Standards

Focus	Minimum Data Set	Description
Who	Patient/Client	Person receiving service
What	Event	Service received
Whom	Human Resources	Person providing service
How much	Financial	Service cost
Where	Organization	Service location

◆━━━◆

FIGURE 10.1. Framework for data standards in 1989. (Adapted from Leginski WA, Croze C, et al. *Data Standards for Mental Health Decision Support Systems*, 1989.)

mum content needed to facilitate mental health program management as well as the basic guideline for the system needed to collect and report this information in a way that is useful in making decisions. However, the organization and financing of mental health and substance abuse care (behavioral health care) has undergone tremendous changes since the FN 10 report was published in 1989. The MHSIP community has initiated a number of task forces including an FN 11 task force to facilitate enrollment tracking, include encounter and performance indicator data, and address the special needs of children. Recognizing the need to take a person-centered approach, MHSIP's efforts have included the design and implementation of a consumer-oriented report card, consumer outcomes measures, and system performance indicators.[3–5]

The MHSIP data standards provide an excellent foundation for the information systems currently required by managed behavioral health care. The new Decision Support 2000+ effort builds on and expands these MHSIP efforts by including the health status of the population, enrollment, encounter and outcome data, as well as system description and performance information[6] (Fig. 10.2).

Today's Mandate

The need for information versus data has expanded exponentially in the managed care era. Dramatic changes are taking place in the roles and types of stakeholders involved in the behavioral healthcare system. These changes have created a need to expand and improve information, and to provide support for decisions made on a daily basis. The quality of information will determine the quality of care; without good data, stakeholders cannot make good decisions and without good decisions, the system cannot continue to operate. This chapter discusses the emerging purpose, features, principles, and data standards for Decision Support 2000+, a newly formed mental health information system for both the public and private sectors.

Information should be available quickly, electronically, and in an easily accessible format. Currently, this situation does not prevail in the mental health field because of dramatic underinvestment in modern information systems and lack of application of modern information technology to mental health problems.

Such information should also be confidential, protect personal privacy, be available for consumer review and correction, and be used only for medical purposes to improve personal well-being. Currently, this situation does not exist in the mental health field because medical records are fragmented, maintained on paper, transmitted through facsimile machines, sent electronically over the Internet without protection, and available for commercial exploitation.

The mental health field (and, indeed, the human service system as a whole) needs standardized data to manage care effectively. The field also requires measures to evaluate the quality of the care provided, with respect to both practices and outcomes. No widely accepted clinical or system guidelines exist with which to standardize practice or to provide criteria for judging provider and system performance. Availability of data systems for collecting this information in a uniform and comparable way will enable communication among participants and across systems of care.

Today's technology makes possible a revolution in information: multiple users can participate in what is virtually a *single information system* that will enable them to share data and communicate effectively. If they adhere to established standards for data collection, this virtual system can be used to meet their information needs, whether they are consumers or providers making choices about

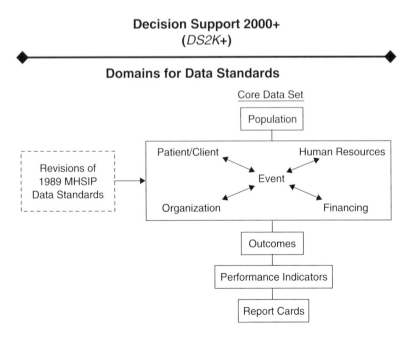

FIGURE 10.2. Framework for data standards in Decision Support 2000+.

treatments, payers deciding among health plans, managers allocating financial and human resources, or researchers determining the need for services in a community. This can be accomplished while protecting the privacy and confidentiality of personal medical records.

To be useful in the current environment, mental health information needs to span from population characteristics through the effects of services. The Survey and Analysis Branch within the Center for Mental Health Services (CMHS) is currently supporting work to develop the framework for such a system. Support and buy-in from all major stakeholders in the system is critical to the success of these projects. To this end, CMHS is working with Abt Associates, the National Association of State Mental Health Program Directors (NASMHPD), MHSIP, and a broad array of expert consultants from major stakeholder groups, such as mental health consumers, family members, the managed behavioral healthcare industry, individual service providers, payers, researchers, and experts in mental health electronic records and information technology.

Decision Support 2000+

Purpose

To respond to the mental health field's lack of standardized data, uniform measures, and an accessible and effective information system, the CMHS project team is developing data standards, minimum data recording requirements, procedures, and an information system for mental health services. These activities build on what the field has already accomplished, using resources currently in place and focusing on areas that need further work. Decision Support 2000+ is being designed to do the following:

Improve decisions: Clinical and administrative decisions made by consumers and family members, providers, payers, managers, and researchers will be enhanced by an information system that provides all the data needed, quickly, accurately, and efficiently.
Improve services: An information system that makes available to stakeholders reliable data on a community's mental health needs, services, service users, costs, revenues, performance, and outcomes is critical to improving care.
Improve accountability: To be most beneficial, information on accountability needs to be readily available within the framework of continuous quality improvement.
Improve communications: Effective communication within the mental health system as well as between it and other human service systems is essential for delivering quality care.

A group of experts and stakeholders was convened to guide the development of Decision Support 2000+ and to address the goals identified above. This group recommended that the information system should be able to

- span the entire mental health system, from epidemiology, to service delivery, to outcomes;
- link with information systems in a broad range of agencies, locations, programs, organization;
- meet the needs of all relevant groups, including consumers, families, providers, payers, managed care organizations, state mental health agencies, administrators, researchers, policy makers, and advocates;
- make use of modern technology while ensuring privacy and confidentiality of data;
- be flexible enough to incorporate information and assessment tools that measure the cultural competence of services; and
- facilitate clinical and organizational decision making and enhance the quality of care.

Description

Decision Support 2000+ contains four categories of data: descriptive, prescriptive, evaluative, and corrective. Each type of information has its value for addressing particular types of questions:

Descriptive information: What are we doing?
Prescriptive information: What should we be doing?
Evaluative information: How well are we doing?
Corrective information: How do we improve?

Figures 10.3 and 10.4 illustrate the Decision Support 2000+ model. Figure 10.3 summarizes the key information modules (see descriptions below) and shows how they can be linked together and transformed to answer a range of critical stakeholder questions. The key information modules are

- population, plan enrollment, encounters with service providers, and the financial, organizational, and human resource characteristics of clinical and administrative entities within the care system;
- measures that reflect adherence to system and clinical guidelines; and
- results reported through system performance measures, consumer outcome measures, and surveys of consumers, providers, and others.

Figure 10.4, by contrast, shows how both the mental health care system and Decision Support 2000+ are linked to the care and information systems of other human service agencies. The stakeholders in the behavioral healthcare system provide data for and receive information from Decision Support 2000+. Stakeholder queries can range from questions about plan quality to questions about adherence to practice guidelines.

The information system records data from various sources that are needed to manage mental health systems effectively. Population data describe demographic characteristics, medical and mental health status, and level of functioning, as well as quality of life of community members. Enrollment data describe demographic,

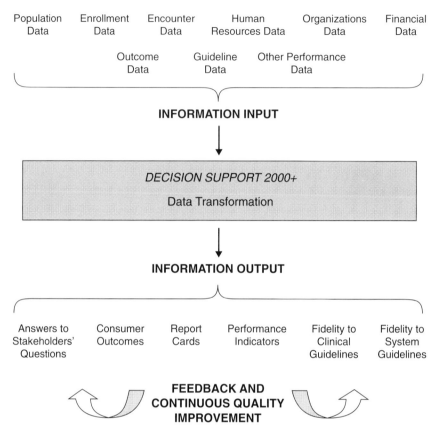

FIGURE 10.3. Quality improvement cycle in public sector behavioral health.

insurance, and baseline health and mental health status of enrollees and their family members. Encounter data characterize all users of services (e.g., health and mental health status, diagnosis, symptoms, functional status, etc.), types of services used, and frequency of use. Financial data reflect costs of services, administrative costs, other expenditures, and revenues. Human resource data describe the characteristics of providers of care, support staff, and other personnel. Information about organizational structure and process is reflected by organizational data.

Clinical guideline data serve three primary functions: clinical decision support (selection of the most effective treatments for conditions), treatment process tracking (a detailed and standardized record of clinical interventions), and guideline variance tracking (the congruence between guideline-recommended treatment and actual treatment delivered). While significant progress has been made in establishing the importance of clinical guidelines and their measures, guidelines are currently unavailable for many disorders. There is no consensus on which guidelines are the best, and few clinicians have been trained in their use;

Decision Support 2000+ in Context

Sources and Users of Data

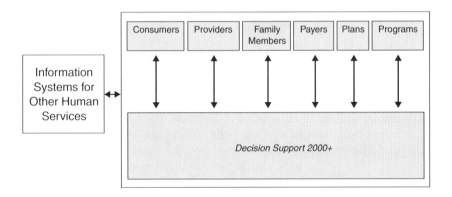

FIGURE 10.4. Framework for flow of data between systems and users.

clinical guidelines software has only recently become available. Implementation of measures for treatment process and guideline variance tracking systems awaits a standard terminology of treatments with associated definitions and codes that can be integrated into routinely used software. Clinical decision support, in turn, depends on building interfaces with treatment process tracking and consumer characteristics. As we develop this component of Decision Support 2000+, we will involve end-users in the development of guidelines, taxonomies, measures, and software so that they are meaningful, reputable, and user-friendly.

Even though system guideline data are essential for improving the quality of care and efficiency of operations, they are only in the earliest stages of development. They specify measures with respect to infrastructure, executive, and management functions; service components directly operated; and service functions outside of mental health that support clinical programs. Prototypical system guidelines and measures exist in several locations, including the National Alliance for the Mentally Ill's recently published manual on the Program for Assertive Community Treatment (PACT);[7] operational manuals prescribing organizational practices (accreditation, credentialing, personnel and financial management, buildings maintenance); clinical interventions (involuntary commitment, seclusion, and restraint); and the quality improvement tools used by some state mental health agencies for assessing provider and organizational performance. The area of system guidelines is being defined and clarified for the first time through the work of the CMHS project team. As minimum data sets are developed, we will also clarify the measurement of system guidelines.

Performance indicators, report cards, and consumer outcome data are critical for the accountability, quality improvement, and management of mental health systems. Although the field lacks uniform sets of performance indicators and outcome measures, there is an emerging consensus on the critical components for each, and steady progress toward standardization. Several initiatives are under way to standardize measures and definitions across systems, to develop methodological and implementation guidelines, and to analyze, interpret, and present results in comparable ways.

Key Features

Decision Support 2000+ has several hallmark features: protection of privacy and confidentiality of personal medical records, evolution of field-wide standards for data recording, reliance on existing information whenever possible to reduce the cost of implementing the new system, and the linkage of data from different sources using Internet-based query technology.

Protecting Privacy and Confidentiality

Decision Support 2000+ is being designed to protect privacy and confidentiality of personal medical records using modern information technology. An overarching concern in conceptualizing the new system was the need to specifically address these issues throughout the development and implementation process. In preparing the requirements analysis for Decision Support 2000+,[6] a document was commissioned regarding the issue of privacy from the consumer point of view. This document is available as part of the requirements analysis on the Web site, *www.mhsip.org*.

Privacy and confidentiality are of concern to most people. Stigma, loss of control, exploitation, and potential negative consequences are concerns that become magnified when considering medical records, and mental health records in particular. Such considerations have provided strong motivation for passage of a healthcare bill of rights giving consumers the ability to gain access to medical records and correct errors in them. The bill would also bring forces together to promote human rights preservation and enhancement through better privacy and confidentiality protections.

In mental health, human rights and dignity are basic values. Any effort to address privacy and confidentiality must start with human values and ethics. Hence, these values must provide a foundation for any work undertaken in this area. In recognition of this, the Workgroup for the Computerization of Behavioral Health and Human Services Records[8] has designed a virtual medical record for behavioral health care in which the key to the medical record is controlled by the consumer. This proposed virtual record is also based on technology that makes it feasible to protect privacy and to control confidentiality. Decision Support 2000+ will incorporate the fundamental concepts elaborated by the workgroup.

The U.S. Department of Health and Human Services is currently developing federal regulations to protect privacy and confidentiality of medical records. Monitoring developments within these regulations is needed with respect to their potential impact on behavioral health care, particularly in mental health. Thus, the regulations ultimately released by the department will provide another element of the foundation for Decision Support 2000+.

Establishing Standards

Decision Support 2000+ recommends standards for data recording that permit information reporting at the person, health plan, local, state, and national levels, including minimum data sets, measures and instruments, and procedures for collecting and analyzing data. It builds on the work of MHSIP in developing standards for mental health. MHSIP created a task force in the late 1980s to review existing data standards and recommend revisions. The task force presented minimum data sets for patient/client, event/encounter, human resources, financial and organization data in its 1989 report, *Data Standards for Mental Health Decision Support Systems* (FN-10).[2] Subsequently, recommendations were made regarding data elements relevant to children.[5] Thanks to the quality of MHSIP's work, all states have now voluntarily adopted many of these standards. The updating and refining of FN-10[3] is being continued through the development of Decision Support 2000+ and elaboration of minimum data sets for each of its components.

Using Existing Data

Decision Support 2000+ makes use of existing information technology and data collection activities and allows users to bring their current practices closer to their ideal without major overhauls and massive investments. It would be impossible to build, implement, and finance Decision Support 2000+ de novo. Most components of the system already exist in one form or another. The federal and some state governments collect population-level data; managed behavioral healthcare organizations and providers collect enrollment, encounter, and outcome data, use financial and human resource data, and report on performance indicators. Measures are currently being developed for clinical and system guidelines because of the rapid evolution of this field. We need to expand and standardize these data collection efforts, but should not minimize how much exists. The issue is one of reaching a consensus on how to improve on what we have, not on rebuilding.

The same is true for information systems. Clearly, problems exist with incompatibility in hardware and software; systems that cannot communicate with one another cannot share information. But the Internet is an untapped resource, and advances in data warehousing and object-oriented technologies are enabling us to overcome local differences. Other technical issues must be resolved; we need unique identifiers to link data concerning people, programs, or plans from different databases. We need dependable ways to ensure privacy and confidentiality; we need to be able to collect comparable information in an efficient and affordable way. Again, the issue is one of improvement and consensus, not starting over.

Linking Data

Part of the enormous potential of Decision Support 2000+ lies in its capacity to link data from different sources, both within the mental health system and between mental health and other service systems. By drawing from several different data sets through an Internet-based query system, it is possible to answer key questions ranging from the outcome of a single individual's treatment to projections of service needs and financing requirements for entire populations.

By virtual linking of data sets, information about persons can be used to improve the quality of care and to evaluate plans and programs. For example, quality of care could be greatly enhanced through the implementation of a virtual integrated patient record spanning the mental health, health, and human services delivery systems.[8] Linking together the enrollment and encounter data aggregated for all persons served by a plan can be used to show whether standards within a contract have been met, such as requirements for providing mental health services to certain percentages and categories of a state's population. Similarly, linking data from consumer satisfaction surveys and other performance measures with aggregated enrollment and encounter data can show the relationship between such factors as satisfaction, availability of specialists, denials of services, and rates of plan enrollment and disenrollment.

The virtual linking of data will meet the following mental health needs:

The need to coordinate care more efficiently and effectively. A primary barrier to competent delivery of mental health and human services is the lack of a coordinated communication system that would allow for the sharing of timely, accurate, and appropriate information among all the agencies and service systems involved in care.

The need to meet reporting requirements. Most mental health organizations are held accountable to public or private payers and are routinely required to report to them. Exchange of core data sets, agreement on data exchange protocols, and use of Web-based Internet and Intranet applications would increase the efficiency and cost-effectiveness of data collection and reporting.

The need for research. Mental health phenomena at both the person and the service levels are enormously complex. Our ability to understand current circumstances and predict future trends depends on our knack for examining the many factors that affect outcomes and performance. This, in turn, depends on being able to link data.

Many challenges exist in linking the components of an information system and then linking that system to others. These include creation of privacy-protected unique client and provider identifiers, linking structurally different databases, and collecting and reporting real-time data. When linking data sets, it is critical that data elements and coding be clearly specified to avoid misunderstanding and unwanted variation in coding items. Data collection procedures and databases that serve multiple purposes, such as reimbursement and quality measurement, are more likely to be adopted by users than more limited ones; this increases the need for instruments that are straightforward and transparent and that minimize additional staff training and development of training materials and documentation.

Status and Next Steps

With guidance from a technical expert workgroup, the CMHS project team has completed the requirements analysis for Decision Support 2000+. For each component, this analysis describes the field's achievements and remaining work in terms of the degree of consensus that exists on *domains* (issues, categories, or topics of interest), *indicators* (measurable activities, events, characteristics, or items that represent a domain), and *measures* (the instruments used to assess, evaluate, and reflect an indicator); if the measures have been *field tested* and/or *implemented*; and whether the component is fully *ready for inclusion* in the information system. The components are at different levels of development. There is a fairly broad consensus on what to include within the information system for the enrollment and encounter components, for example, but problems such as specifying unique identifiers remain unresolved. For other components, particularly population, financial, and guideline data, much work remains.

The complete requirements analysis is posted on the MHSIP Web site (*www.mhsip.org*) for broad review and comment by the field. For those who do not have the time to review the entire requirements analysis, brief summaries for each component are available on the Web site.

No typology is currently available for organizational and financial arrangements under managed behavioral health care. The team will address this critical gap in our knowledge base and will assess the extent to which the requirements analysis fits each of the major arrangements identified within the typology. This analysis will ensure that Decision Support 2000+, as it is refined, is appropriate for and relevant to the needs of evolving organizational and financial arrangements.

Once the typology is available, the project team will move on to the next phase. Over the next two years, groups of experts will convene and address outstanding issues such as creating unique identifiers, selecting key performance indicators, and recommending uniform outcome measures. They will also develop core minimum data sets for recommendation to the field. While users should collect any data that meet their particular needs, widespread use of the minimum data sets will provide the field with uniform and comparable data to facilitate communication and decision making.

Conclusion

Decision Support 2000+ is an integrated, public health–oriented information system that corresponds with the current and future information needs of the mental health field. Implementation of this information system will facilitate the availability of comparable data to the field for decision support for planning, service design, clinical feedback, and evaluation. Widespread use of the information system will be of tremendous benefit to the entire mental health community.

References

1. Patton RE, Leginski WA. *The Design and Content of a National Mental Health Statistics System.* National Institute of Mental Health, Series FN no. 8. DHHS publ. no. (ADM) 83-1095. Washington, DC: NIMH, 1983.
2. Leginski WA, Croze C, Driggers J, et al. *Data Standards for Mental Health Decision Support Systems.* National Institute of Mental Health, Series FN no. 10. DHHS publ. no. (ADM) 89-1589. Washington, DC: NIMH, 1989.
3. MHSIP Ad Hoc Group. *The Handbook of Mental Health Data—A Reference Manual for Anyone Who Wants to Collect, Find, Report, Understand or Use Mental Health Data.* Draft 5/23/97. Rockville, MD: Center for Mental Health Services, 1997.
4. MHSIP Report Card Phase II Task Force. *The MHSIP Consumer-Oriented Mental Health Report Card.* Rockville, MD: Center for Mental Health Services, 1996.
5. MHSIP Task Force on Enhancing MHSIP to Meet the Needs of Children. *Enhancing MHSIP to Meet the Needs of Children—Final Report.* Rockville, MD: Center for Mental Health Services, 1992.
6. Minden SL, Davis S, Ganju V, et al. Draft requirements analysis for Decision Support 2000+. *www.mhsip.org,* 2000.
7. Allness DJ, Knoedler WH. *The PACT Model of Community-Based Treatment for Persons with Severe and Persistent Mental Illness. A Manual for PACT Startup.* Arlington VA: NAMI, 1998.
8. Workgroup for the Computerization of Behavioral Health and Human Services Records. *The Virtual Consumer and Family-Focused Behavioral Health and Human Services Record.* Prepared for the Center for Mental Health Services. Rockville, MD: Workgroup for the Computerization of Behavioral Health and Human Services Records, 1998.

Part V
Organizational Issues

Introduction

NANCY M. LORENZI

As the quantity of behavioral health knowledge increased, informatics professionals developed technical tools and strategies to better manage the volume and flow of information. These technical tools and strategies are constantly becoming more sophisticated, thus affecting additional aspects of behavioral healthcare organizations. Unfortunately, their organizational impacts are often not well understood. These impacts and the managerial strategies needed for dealing with the changing world are typically not as easy to define and measure as their more technical counterparts.

It has become rather obvious in recent years that to successfully introduce major new systems into complex organizations requires an effective blend of good technical and organizational skills. The technically "best" system may be woefully inadequate if people with low psychological ownership of that system resist its implementation. On the other hand, people with high ownership can make a technically mediocre system function fairly well.

A wide range of skills is necessary to effectively interface with all of the information system stakeholders. A significant behavioral health informatics project typically impacts a wide range of people: physicians, nurses, other members of the healthcare team, support staff, administrators, patients, and vendors. To ensure success, those who are spearheading the project must be skilled at dealing at both the people or individual level and the organizational or group level. An implementation can only be as successful as its ability to meet the often-conflicting needs of the various stakeholders. It is through these people and organizational skills that the implementers determine these needs, build support for their work, and negotiate solutions to problems and conflicts.

The four chapters in this section focus on organizational issues. Chapter 11 focuses on the "people issues" and reviews the barriers and resistance that a typical organization experiences when implementing new informatics systems. Chapter 12 focuses on leadership, namely the roles and responsibilities of the chief executive officer and the chief information officer. Chapter 13 discusses the overall organizational aspects of applying a new informatics system. Chapter 14 centers on evaluating the impact of the behavioral healthcare system on an organization and its people.

11
Barriers and Resistance to Informatics in Behavioral Health Care

ROBERT T. RILEY, NANCY M. LORENZI, AND NAAKESH A. DEWAN

Susan Harding stood by the coffee machine early one Monday, taking in a mega-dose of caffeine—the traditional drug of choice for computer types. As the project leader for the implementation of the new practice management system for the Gotham Center for Behavioral Health, she was contemplating the typically hectic week ahead. Her thoughts were interrupted by the loud and rather excited voice of Dan St. James, a middle-aged therapist in the practice, talking to someone out in the hall.

"Did you see yesterday's *Gotham Gazette*? Look at this—three articles in just one issue! 'High School Students Change Grades in Local School Computer.' And look at this, 'Security Flaw Found in Popular Internet Program.' And this one, too, 'Chain Stores Tracking and Selling Your Buying Profiles.' My God, they want us to put all our diagnoses and treatment protocols into this new computer system. Why don't we just take out ads in the *Gazette* and publish them!"

"Now come on, Dan, I'm sure it's not going to be all that bad." Susan recognized the voice of Bob Hobbs, one of the oldest members of the practice.

From behind her in the lounge, Susan heard two of the junior members of the practice laughing. "Sounds like the dinosaurs are on the rampage again," one said. "Well, Bob didn't sound too excited," replied the other. "Yes, but he can afford to ignore it. Bob's in the checkout lane anyway; he'll be retired before long. The ones really feeling the pain are the ones like Dan, the dinosaurs who are going to be around for a while and who will have to adapt."

Meanwhile, from out in the hall, Susan heard Dan announcing to Bob that he was going to call for a meeting of the administrative committee "to really look into these security issues."

Susan thought, "Wonderful! That's all I need right now—another meeting to prepare a presentation for. I should have gone into something quiet and peaceful—like lion taming." After pouring another cup of coffee, she trudged back to her office to begin her week with a lot less enthusiasm.

Introducing Informatics Systems into Organizations

The above scenario was constructed from numerous interactions that we have had with people in all areas of health care, who are seeing the healthcare arena that they have known, loved, and mastered changing rapidly and dramatically before their eyes. While a new information system may be straightforward in a technical sense, we have to implement these new systems within complex organizations composed of equally complex individuals. It is often said that the only person that welcomes change is a wet baby. Changes within organizations very commonly engender significant resistance.

One of our major concerns is that it is easy to listen to the words of the Dans among us and take their statements literally, which can often be very misleading. Whenever we talk about resistance to change, we must ensure that we have correctly identified the change(s) being resisted. This chapter discusses resistance to change and organizational strategies to overcome resistance.

The following four categories of resistance are often useful in analyzing specific situations:

Resistance to environmental changes—changes in the organization's general environment that will have impact on the way that the organization functions and possibly on its very survival.

Resistance to general organizational or systems changes—changes in the way the organization is structured or the broad systems that it uses to pursue its mission. These changes might result from either external or internal forces.

Resistance to the changers—it matters little what the change is. "If 'they' are for it, I am against it!"

Resistance to specific changes—changes such as a new or updated computer system, which is resisted based on its own merit or the process by which it is implemented.

If we do not accurately identify the real source of the resistance, we can waste a lot of time, money, and staff goodwill by using inappropriate solutions to the real problem. For example, high-quality training on how to use a new system can be a tool to combat the fourth type of resistance, but it will do little good against the first three.

The relevance to today's behavioral medicine area is obvious. As the lead paragraph in a recent *Wall Street Journal* article stated, "The old reality for many psychiatrists was a private practice filled with long-term patients who paid $100 or more for 50 minutes of talk. The new reality? Managing medications for up to 30 new patients a week for half the hourly fee—and answering to case managers who aren't even doctors."[1] People facing stressful changes induced by powerful environmental forces such as managed care are going to seek targets they feel they *can* fight, and a new computer system is often an attractive target of opportunity.

The management lesson is this—identify and fight the real problem first. If the real problem is resistance to what is happening in health care, deal with the problem at that level first.

Levels of Resistance

The levels of resistance to a new informatics system can vary widely both between and among specific groups. Resistance can involve a less-than-enthusiastic response, a refusal to participate in training, an organized protest among colleagues, or sabotage of the system through acts of either omission or commission. Incidentally, such sabotage is more common than often realized.

The aim of effective change management techniques is not to eliminate all resistance. This is typically impossible when a group of workers is involved. The aims are (1) to keep initial general resistance at reasonable levels, (2) to prevent that initial resistance from growing to serious levels, and (3) to identify and deal with any pockets of serious resistance that do occur despite the previous efforts. Unfortunately for the healthcare industry, many consultants are making a good living from solving implementation crises that could have been reasonably prevented at the early stages.

Confidentiality as a Stalking Horse

In the behavioral area, concerns about confidentiality are both real and serious. The potential for patient harm is tremendous.[2] Yet, confidentiality has also been a definite stalking horse for those resisting computer systems in the healthcare area. Confidentiality can never be an absolute, and it is unreasonable to hold new systems to standards never achieved by the systems traditionally in place. Healthcare professionals must insist that both the computerized and noncomputerized systems with which they interact are designed and operated with high but realistic standards of confidentiality.

Acceptance of Accountability

The healthcare area has been fortunate that managed care developed so slowly. The stresses currently being undergone affected most professions several years earlier. For a variety of reasons, society is unwilling to trust its professionals in the way it did in the past. Therefore, society is demanding accountability, which in turn means measurability. As a result, the introduction of new computerized systems often raises the specter of increased measurement and increased supervision by those paying the bills. This is a reality, but the information system is merely implementing it, not causing it.

Why Physicians Resist Informatics

Resistance to change in healthcare organizations is not limited to physicians; however, their dominant role makes their resistance especially telling. Physicians have readily accepted many changes in the practice of medicine over the past fifty years such as the use of new medical devices, new drugs, and new surgical procedures. Why, then, is informatics so commonly resisted? Any major new system is going to generate reasonable amounts of the FUD factor—fear, uncertainty, and doubt. However, here are some specific reasons that are quite relevant to physician resistance to informatics:

Perceived low personal benefits: Physicians often perceive, whether rightly or wrongly, that the informatics system will have little positive impact on making their job easier or improving patient care—two of their major concerns.

Fear of loss of status: If the proposed system involves activities such as direct physician order entry, the physicians may perceive a loss of status in doing data entry as opposed to "barking out" orders for others to implement. In addition, tersely worded system-generated "alerts" can be an assault on the professionals' egos.

Fear of revealing ignorance: The computer represents a completely new area of knowledge to many physicians and an area in which they may not be confident of their learning skills. To these physicians, accustomed to being viewed as assertive sources of knowledge, the informatics area can be perceived as a potential source of embarrassment, especially if lesser mortals appear more proficient.

Fear of an imposed discipline: Many clinical systems impose a lack of flexibility that makes physicians feel that their needs, desires, and historic procedures are being made secondary to the "needs" of the new system. Through the intentional limitation of choices, physicians may be forced into the use of only "approved" protocols.

Fear of wasted time: Physicians are notoriously time-conscious and tend to resist the training or learning time necessary to become comfortable with informatics systems. In addition, they are highly sensitive to time required to use the system and are not necessarily charitable in judging whether the new system takes more or less time than previous methods. The prospect of long-run benefits may well not outweigh the perception of reduced short-run efficiencies.

Fear of unwanted accountability: Even those with a limited understanding of informatics realize that modern systems accumulate significant databases that can be used to analyze the activities of individual system users. Those accustomed to being held accountable on only a few broad measures often fear the creation of an environment in which their performance can be quickly and easily monitored on a wide range of variables. At a more dramatic level, increased measurement and data raise the specter of potential increases in legal liability.[3]

Fear of new demands: A subtle and often unrecognized fear is a concern about what new informatics systems will do to the accustomed and comfortable ways in which physicians fill their time. One of the impacts of informatics on other professions has been that computerized systems have increasingly assumed the burden of the routine, freeing the professional for the more complex and creative aspects of the professional role.

The breadth of the above concerns shows how difficult the problem of overcoming physician resistance can be. When dealing with a group of physicians all of the above concerns can appear in varying combinations among individuals within the group.

Key Organizational Strategies

The realities of managed care are forcing most behavioral health organizations to sharply upgrade their computer systems. As this occurs, several organizational strategies can smooth the implementation process. In theory, these strategies should be unnecessary with people trained in the behavioral areas. However, experience has taught us that organizations of behaviorally trained people typically suffer from the "shoemaker's children" syndrome in terms of their internal operations.

These following strategies have proven effective for us in many situations[4]:

Collecting Benchmark Data

One of the first steps in preparing to implement a new system is to gather accurate performance data for the existing system(s). A common form of resistance to a new system is the making of constant unfavorable comparisons to the old system. While presenting factual data will not overcome emotional reactions, it is important that unfounded allegations about the new system not go unanswered.

Analyzing the Benefits

Early in the overall process, an accurate cost/benefit analysis must be performed from the viewpoint of the physician users—and other major user groups as well. A very valid question for any user is, "What's in it for me?" If the answer is, "Nothing," then why should the user embrace the system? This situation typically calls for a rethinking of the overall system design to ensure that there are some benefits for all the affected groups.

General Organizational Climate

If the general organizational climate is relatively negative, attack that problem directly with sound organizational development techniques. Installing an informatics system, no matter how good it may be, will not solve this problem. In fact, the system may be doomed by the negative general climate.

Background Education

This is where the broader issues raised above must be addressed in a straight-forward manner. Why is the system needed? How will confidentiality standards be maintained? What will the system be able to measure over time? How will these measurements be used? Who will have access to what information? People are entitled to answers to these questions if we expect their support. Moreover, people at all levels of the organization must be educated in this way, not just the clinical staff.

Potential Champions

An informatics system needs champions. The optimal approach is to identify several medically respected physicians to fulfill this champion role. They should be integrated into the planning process from the beginning, with their advice sought on virtually all aspects of the development and implementation process.

A potentially useful—but also potentially dangerous—group is the subset of physicians that we call the "techie-docs." These are the computer enthusiasts who often consider themselves experts in medical informatics, despite having relatively spotty knowledge in the area. This group can easily cause two types of problems: (1) they may advocate inappropriate or infeasible proposals that sound good to other physicians who know even less about informatics, and (2) they may not be that respected in an overall sense but keep getting appointed as the physician representatives to informatics committees. This is why we stress that informatics systems must have some champions who are *respected medically*.

General Ownership

Developing respected champions is only the first step in building general ownership in the system. The primary twin tools for general ownership are involvement and communication. The single best tool in building ownership is participation in the overall process—planning, design, selection, and implementation—by those whom the new system will affect. However, there is an important issue that arises in medical areas. In systems of any size, the participation often has to be representative rather than total.

Modern rapid-prototyping software development tools are an excellent means of developing ownership. Various groups can be shown rough system prototypes, and their inputs can be rapidly incorporated in successive stages of the prototype. Some minor changes can often be made "before their very eyes!"

A common problem is that once the prototyping is done, a black hole develops in an information sense. The users became relatively excited about the project and then—nothing! It is important that they be kept aware that work is rapidly progressing on the system. It may be useful even to stage some brief presentations by the developers to highlight their progress.

Building Ownership

The danger is that the participation process often attracts the amateur techies in the organization, either by self-selection or by appointment. However, these people may not be high-clout people in the organization. It is critical to have some participation from key power people. In healthcare organizations, this often translates as people who are highly respected *clinically*.

Rapid Implementation

As indicated above, a potential downside of involving people early to build ownership is the waiting period between the early involvement and the actual implementation. Within reason, it is a good strategy to concentrate resources on a limited number of projects to minimize the waiting period for system implementation. This will lessen the efforts needed to rebuild the ownership developed in earlier stages.

Realistic Expectations

No matter how good the new informatics system is, it will not improve the quality of the coffee. If the physicians are oversold on what the new system will do, the system is doomed to be regarded as at least a partial failure. This includes setting realistic expectations for the impacts on initial productivity during the early implementation stages. It is almost inevitable that productivity will initially decline, no matter how good the system and the preparations for its implementation.

Timely, Appropriate Training

Getting physicians to participate in informatics training in a traditional classroom sense is notoriously difficult. Any training must be brief, high quality, closely timed to the point of need, and specifically directed to the physicians' needs. Extra sessions will need to be held to pick up the stragglers. Part of the training will have to be accomplished hands-on through the support process. Ego issues can also be important, especially for senior people who may be anxious about their lack of computer abilities. Private or small-group sessions often help considerably in these cases. Similarly, the style, pace, and depth of training may need to be adjusted for all the various user subgroups. Those doing the training should have outgoing, positive personalities. Good training does more than merely build skills. Ideally, education starts the selling process, participation adds enthusiasm, and training is the final opportunity to "close the sale."

Quality training can help significantly in reducing the staff's anxieties about using a new system. However, the timing is critical. Training that is either too early or too late will waste resources and raise frustrations, not alleviate them.

Extensive Support

With modern software tools, there is no excuse for developing systems without extensive contextual on-line user support written in language that the users can understand. Supplementary written support should also be provided in a format most comfortable for the users. For example, physicians might prefer a "cheat sheet" in the 3×5 card format that many use for various purposes.

When the system is first installed, ample on-site help should be available, to be subsequently replaced with good phone support as the initial demands dwindle. Time-conscious physicians demand prompt, high-quality support or they rapidly become discontented with the system.

System Stability

Physicians are busy people. Even if they are willing to invest the time to learn the system, they almost certainly will not be willing to spend the time to relearn the release of the month. Well-crafted software is relatively stable, at least in its user interface, and effective prototyping should sharply limit the number of changes necessary in the interface. There will be bugs, but correcting them should not require constantly modifying the user interface.

Protecting Professional Egos

Although it is costly, skilled one-on-one or small-group training may be an effective strategy for those physicians and other professionals most likely to be affected by computer phobia. This is especially important if these particular professionals are also highly respected medically by their peers within the organization.

Professionals have an understandable need for respect. Therefore, the dialogues present in informatics systems should be carefully reviewed for usefulness, clarity, and respectful tone. For example, alerts should be programmed as respectful questions rather than as terse declarative statements. Error messages must give useful instructions for correcting the situation. While these suggestions may sound simple, they are often violated by informatics personnel who are used to functioning under another paradigm of human/computer interface.

Feedback Processes

Any aggressive change management strategy should contain multiple mechanisms for actively soliciting feedback at all stages of the change process. The alternative is to have rumors, half-truths, and even untruths flooding the grapevine. When feedback is solicited and obtained, it must be processed promptly and return feedback provided. Not every issue can be resolved to everyone's satisfaction. This is life in the real world. Still, people must feel that both they and their concerns are regarded as important.

Having Fun

Smart change managers try to introduce an element of fun into the change management process whenever possible. Two techniques that we have seen used numerous times to stimulate the introduction of new clinical systems are lunch-time or end-of-day sessions with free pizza and soft drinks and sessions that feature some nonthreatening competition between the physicians and the system or between physicians using the system and physicians not using the system. The message is that facing the future doesn't have to be grim!

Summary

Experience tells us that motivated, involved people can make bad systems work. After all, they have done it for years. In the same way, unmotivated—or even worse, negatively motivated—people can bring the best system to its knees. Which situation will we have? How well we carry out the steps outlined above will often answer that question.

References

1. Hymowitz C. High anxiety: In the name of Freud, why are psychiatrists complaining so much? *Wall Street Journal* 1995 (December 21):A1.
2. Edwards HB. Managed care and confidentiality. *Behav Health Manag* 1995;15(6): 25–27.
3. Lorenzi NM, Riley RT, Ball MJ, Douglas JV. *Transforming Health Care Through Information: Case Studies.* New York: Springer-Verlag, 1995.
4. Lorenzi NM, Riley RT. *Organizational Aspects of Health Informatics: Managing Technological Change.* New York: Springer-Verlag, 1994.

12
Leadership Roles and Responsibilities of the Chief Executive Officer and Chief Information Officer

NANCY M. LORENZI, ROBERT T. RILEY, AND NAAKESH A. DEWAN

Computerized information systems in behavioral health care have existed since the 1960s.[1] The first systems were mainly administrative patient data systems, which were followed by the development of computer systems to support clinical processes. Later systems incorporated both functions and were able to provide benefits for both management and clinical levels. Benefits to management include support for planning and allocating of resources, clinical audit, and outcome measurement.[2] At the clinical level information systems can support the coordination of services, patient assessment, treatment plans, and reviews, and provide a basis for continuity of care.[3] Despite the early introduction of such systems and potential benefits, the diffusion of information technology in this area has been slow.[4] The diffusion of technology in behavioral health began to increase in the 1990s.

Regardless of the size of the organization or when the diffusion of information technology came or will come, two people can be identified as the chief executive officer (CEO) and the chief information officer (CIO), and thus as key people for successful implementation. It is imperative that these two people understand the vision for the use of informatics to support the clinical and administrative aspects of the organization. It is also imperative that they work together for a successful implementation and then a successful management of the changed organization. Each person has a different set of organizational roles, but their respective roles must be complementary and easily understood by all in the organization. This chapter provides an in-depth perspective on the roles of the CEO and CIO in a behavioral healthcare organization. For some organizations, the CEO and the CIO will be the same person; for others a database programmer or statistician will serve as the de facto CIO. (In behavioral healthcare organizations, the CEO is often called the "executive director," especially in nonprofit human service organizations.) In either case it is essential to formalize and systematize the roles, responsibilities, and activities of these positions in the contemporary behavioral healthcare organization.

Chief Executive Officer

Today's CEO possesses talents such as financial acumen, strategic thinking, communication abilities, personal insight, boundless energy, understanding, cross-industry experience, and diverse interpersonal skills. CEOs focus on the big picture and the broader perspective so as to responsibly lead the ever more diversified work force.[5] The CEO has overall responsibility for formulating policy, and is generally assisted by senior management in formulating and implementing policies, controls, and limits to ensure that the risks of derivative activities and the manner in which they are conducted are in accordance with the board's authorization.

The primary job of a CEO is the long-term viability of the organization's business. This visionary leadership is achieved by communicating the vision that leads to a shared purpose for the entire organization. CEOs are strategic visionaries and they must perceive the big picture and persuade people to share their vision, trust them, and follow them. For many CEOs, the ability to lead is instinctive. CEOs look to their boards for advice and input in the evaluation of ideas, financial situations, and action plans. CEOs also confer with company management for viability and feedback. CEOs research the impact—financial, social, psychological—of the strategic vision, listening carefully to responses from employees, customers, board members, and the community.

The success of an organization and the success of a CEO rests heavily upon the leader's abilities to execute his or her strategic vision both in times of calm and in times of crisis. Informed, optimistic, well spoken, and charismatic, the CEO provides stability through motivation and reassurance. CEOs must be consistent and shining examples of the culture they espouse, providing a proactive, focused, and visionary leadership now and into the future.[6]

The CEO also has financial responsibilities that are beyond the role of the chief financial officer. Some of those responsibilities include (1) networking in the financial community, (2) interacting with accountants and lawyers, (3) developing strategies and policies to maintain a strong balance sheet, and (4) continual look for new sources of revenue.

The CEO is also responsible for business strategy and planning, developing new business, and building the company's market share. It is usually in this realm of business strategy that the information systems and informatics issues arise.

As a primary responsibility of today's CEOs, strategic thinking is a central theme in their day-to-day operations. Strategic thinking is the basis for the company's mission and business plan. The CEO's responsibilities—communication with the shareholders and boards, sharing of the company's vision, facilitation of organizational interaction, management of growth, and public relations—all require thoughtful planning and careful articulation.

CEOs today have traded the role of autocrat for the role of strategic liaison. The CEO as the visionary link or conduit between the organization and every individual or group of individuals with whom the CEO interacts, both inside the organization and within the community, provides a continual and convincing sense of purpose, style, and vision.

CEOs need to make sure that their organizations are not only technology friendly but also leaders in the use of technology in every dimension of their business. It is the CEO's job to lead that effort in conjunction with the chief information officer.

As the CEO's visionary, strategic, and leadership role continues its evolution into the 21st century, the CEO will face numerous challenges. CEOs will have to expand their skills to increase their role in the global marketplace and will steadily withdraw from less strategic aspects of business operations. Interpersonal skills will continue to emerge as critical to work-force satisfaction and, consequently, company performance. The advent of information technology will take new shape and present new opportunities. In addition, evolving CEOs, maximizing these opportunities, will continue to create innovative business strategies to keep their organization at the leading competitive edge.

Chief Information Officer

The CIO must focus on the information systems and informatics to ensure that they support the direction of the parent organization. Key CIO processes are necessary for any successful organization. The details and emphasis of these processes may differ between the public and the private sector, but the basic tenets are applicable to any CIO.

A CIO has seven main areas of responsibility: (1) business process analysis and improvement, (2) information resources management/systems development (purchase or build), (3) capital information technology (IT) investment control, (4) performance measurement, (5) IT training/education/communication, (6) strategic and capital planning, and (7) administration.

Business Process Analysis and Improvement

One key role of informatics in a behavioral healthcare setting is to improve the business process and thereby allow the clinical processes to take precedence. The CIO must be part of all business redesign processes in which informatics is a strategic factor in the improvement of direct patient care. The business redesign process is especially important is behavioral health care as e-commerce, e-therapy, and e-managed care become more prevalent.

Information Resources Management/Systems Development (Purchase or Build)/ IT Architecture

Clinicians must be involved in the vision of what needs to happen in a clinical informatics setting. However, it is the CIO who will analyze the organization's information technology architecture and determine if what is needed can be purchased or if it must be built to meet the specific needs of the organization. The

CIO establishes IT policies and standards that promote a secure architecture to support the scientific, engineering, and administrative data and information technology requirements. Access to computers and proximity to ancillary resources, such as the phone, are other issues that pertain to work practice.

Capital IT Investment Control

The capital investment for informatics efforts and information technology must follow the above-mentioned efforts. The organization must decide whether to have an application service provider (ASP) model, have a completely internally run and operated local area network, or have a combination of both. From an informatics perspective, the ASP model allows someone else to manage all mission-critical financial, clinical, and office management functions including internal e-mail, word processing, and calendar management. This complete outsourcing of all IT activities is only beginning to be used by businesses outside of health care and may find a home in behavioral healthcare organizations, which are less capable of raising capital for technology expenses and may be served best with outsourcing everything. This will happen when healthcare organizations recognize that IT is a utility function akin to heat and electricity. Then behavioral healthcare organizations will have to purchase new personal computers, printers, networking equipment every two to three years, and upgrade office and healthcare-specific applications every one to two years. This requirement to keep up with hardware, networking, and software refinements will exact a financial drain on the organization if long-term planning is not conducted. Hardware could represent half of the yearly IT budget.

Performance Measurement

Performance measurement processes must be created to measure not only the IT infrastructure itself in terms of performance standards, but also the contribution of the IT infrastructure and systems to overall mission performance. One role of the CIO is to use key metrics to measure the performance and effectiveness of the IT infrastructure and its contribution to meeting the agency's vision and mission performance. The metrics are intended to quickly convey information that can be acted upon by the CIO. It should be noted that while some IT activities may be program driven, the CIO should introduce and inculcate the key metrics into the program.

Key metrics include the following:

• IT business value—identification of value drivers (internal perspective), customer satisfaction surveys, and interview programs that actively seek out users to determine the level of satisfaction with the products and services provided by the organization.

• Process improvement rate—implementation and application of structured processes, and information system asset base, including the current size in dollars, location, and number of installed components, their remaining useful life, the cost of replacement or substitution, and how IT is changing in size from year to year.

IT Training/Education/Communication

Educating the CEO as well as others in the organization is another responsibility of the CIO. The executive management and staff must be educated on the potential contributions, limitations, and subsequent actual measured performance of IT in accomplishing the critical organizational mission. The CIO must convince the organization's executive management that IT is an essential agent of transformation, help to create a shared vision for this transformation, identify core IT competencies to support the new vision, achieve approval for an overall strategy to achieve these competencies, keep the organization informed of relevant technology trends and the best practices in applying these technologies, and clearly communicate how IT strategies and architecture will be aligned with the new business vision.

Adequate and appropriate training is an important consideration when implementing a new system.[7,8] Robins and Rigby[7] discuss the utilization of key persons to train staff in using new computer systems. Formal training is one aspect of learning a new system, but staff members also need to be given time to learn how to use the system. The limitations of the training process underscores the importance of effective communications to staff about events such as installation and training and more general communication about the project. Such communication is likely to encourage the feeling of involvement of the staff and to facilitate the adoption and ownership of the new technology.[9]

User acceptance[10] and user satisfaction have been strongly linked to the level of user participation in system development. Lack of involvement is likely to lower user acceptance and decrease user satisfaction. On the other hand, users are also more likely to accept a system that they perceive to be useful.

User resistance is common in the medical sphere, and physicians have generally been slow to adopt computerized systems in the healthcare sector.[6] This resistance has been attributed to direct data entry taking too much time, apprehension about changing work patterns, and perceived threats to professional values. The literature in the mental health field refers to these issues as well as concerns about security and confidentiality, being monitored (accountable), and "the dehumanization of the traditional patient/therapist relationship."[2] Recognizing direct benefits is one way of overcoming this resistance.[6]

Strategic and Capital Planning

Budgeting and strategic planning go hand in hand. This aspect of the CIO's job is vital if information is to become a strategic resource for the organization. Moreover, external environmental assessment of available technologies and applications, combined with an assessment of the individuals of the organization, is the first step. Also, the vision and business goals of the organization must be defined. Only then can a true IT strategy be developed. The budgetary impact, as mentioned before, can be significant. The CIO must be very careful not to overstate or understate the value of information technology.

Administration

Overseeing management of IT, including implementing IT acquisition and project management processes, can be the most tiresome of all of the CIO's responsibilities. Very often problems with word processors, replacing the toner cartridge in printers, and other mundane jobs stand in the way of implementing IT systems. IT professionals also tend to be in demand, and employee turnover can be a huge problem. Thus, it is critical to have very rigorous documentation protocols and standard operation procedures in the organization. In the event an employee leaves, one does not have to start over or take months to retrain others.

The responsibilities of the CEO and CIO are intense. In behavioral health care these responsibilities can be assumed by the same person. At times the chief clinical officer or the quality officer assumes the informatics role. Often consultants are required to facilitate IT planning and strategy.

References

1. Sarris A, Sawyer MG. Automated information systems in mental health services: a review. *Int J Mental Health* 1989;8(4):18–30.
2. Glover GR. Mental health care and the big IT. *Psychiatr Bull* 1996;20:195–197.
3. McDougall GM, Adair-Bischoff CE, Grant E. Development of an integrated clinical database system for a regional mental health service. *Psychiatr Serv* 1995;46(8): 826–828.
4. Anderson JG. Clearing the way for physician's use of clinical information systems. *Commun ACM* 1997;40(8):83–90.
5. Greenberg MR. Chief Executive 20th anniversary: Captains Courageous. *Chief Exec* 1997;56.
6. Clark C. "Trust in Me." *Hosp Health Networks* 1996;70(21):36–38.
7. Robins SC, Rigby MJ. Implementing a patient-based information system for the mental health services the importance of a staff focus. In: Lun KC, Degoulet P, Piemme TE, et al, eds. *Medinfo'92 Proceedings of the Seventh World Congress on Medical Informatics, Geneva.* Amsterdam: Elsevier Science, 1992:319–323.
8. Lorenzi NM, Riley RT. *Organizational Aspects of Health Informatics: Managing Technological Change.* New York: Springer-Verlag, 1995.
9. Kaplan B. Reducing barriers to physician entry for computer based patient records. *Top Health Inform Manage* 1994;15(1):24–34.
10. Lorenzi NM, Riley RT, Blyth AJC, Southern G, Dixon BJ. Antecedents of the people and organizational aspects of medical informatics: review of the literature. *JAMIA* 1997;4(2):79–93.

Bibliography

Anderson JG. The business of cyberhealthcare. *MD Comput* 1999;16(6):23–25.

De Graffenried Ruffin M Jr. Many chief information officers will be physician executives. *MD Comput* 1999;16(6):41.

Essex D. Skip the song and dance. *Healthcare Informatics* 1999;16(7):49–56.

Kilbridge PM. E-healthcare—urging providers to embrace the Web. *MD Comput* 2000;17(1):36.

Marietti C. Watch for potholes. *Healthcare Informatics* 2000;17(3):12.

Newell LM, Matthews P. Navigating a CIO Career. *Healthcare Informatics*. 1999;16(11):79–81.

Stead WW. The challenge to health informatics for 1999–2000: form creative partnerships with industry and chief information officers to enable people to use information to improve health. *JAMIA* 1999;6(1):88–89.

13
Organizational Aspects of Implementing Informatics Change

NANCY M. LORENZI AND ROBERT T. RILEY

"Sentimentality will always be man's first revolt against development. [However] the times have made this reaction obsolete. . . . Things are happening so rapidly now that at any moment the present we're living in will be the 'good old days'."[1]

Change is a reality in both our society and our private lives. Our society, professions, and daily work lives are constantly changing at an accelerating rate. Children take for granted the powerful personal computers that we could not even imagine at their age.

The behavioral health professions are undergoing rapid changes, and behavioral health informatics—as part of health informatics in general—is one of the driving forces in that change process. It is impossible to introduce a behavioral health informatics system into an organization without its members feeling its impact. Informatics is all about change—the modification of data into information with eventual evolution into knowledge. Data becomes information only after the data is processed, i.e., altered in ways that make the data useful for decision making. These enhanced decision-making capabilities are inevitably going to affect the organization. Figure 13.1 shows this simple but critical circular relationship between the organization, its informatics systems, and the change process. The organization and its people influence, shape, and alter the nature and use of the informatics systems, which, in turn, influence, shape, and alter the nature, operation, and culture of the organization, and so on.

If we do not manage our change processes, they will manage us—an undesirable outcome. The less control we feel during the change process, the lower our resiliency, that is, our ability to bounce back from the stress of change and our preparation for the inevitable next alteration in today's environment.[2]

Change and Informatics—An Example

At a 1993 conference on the topics of informatics and change, healthcare consultant Bernard Horak presented an example of a professional conflict between nurses and physicians caused by the introduction of a new information technol-

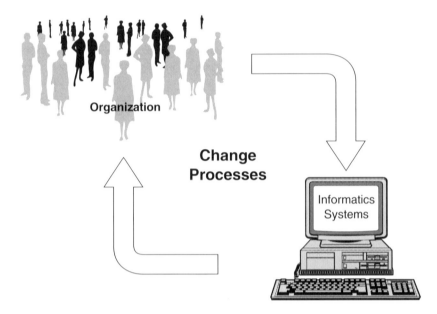

FIGURE 13.1. Circular change relationship between informatics systems, the organizations, and their people.

ogy.[3] In this scenario, adapted by Lorenzi and Riley,[4] the perceived role of nurses as the integrators of patient data/information was challenged when the physicians performed direct order entry into a computer for medications, diagnostics, vital sign monitoring, and so on.

Scenario

The nurse usually serves as an integrator and reviewer when using a manual system on an inpatient unit. The physician expects action after scribbling an order on a piece of paper and giving it to a nurse, unit clerk, or paraprofessional. A nurse typically "cleans it up" and transmits the information or order to the pharmacy, radiology department, laboratory, or dietary department, which will occasionally call the physician back. However, the nurse generally serves as the conduit for the transfer of information. When nurses fill this role, they have a full view of what is happening with the patient as they filter and organize information from various sources. This is a classic work-flow design.

But what happens when the physician is asked to enter orders directly into an information system? In the old system, the physicians issued vague or approximate orders. For example, the physicians would scribble "d.c." or "d/c" for discontinue. They would order "x-rays" and the nurses would figure out that posteroanterior and lateral chest x-rays were wanted. If the physicians tried to enter their orders into the new system as they had in the past, they would either get nothing back or something they did not want. The physicians do not know how to enter an order because they had not actually placed direct orders before. When the physician scribbled an order, the nurse knew the physician, knew exactly what was wanted, and would make it happen. With the new system, this was not possible.

In one hospital, the nurses did not like this new system because they believed that it reduced their role in the overall care process. It took them out of the reviewer, case manager, and integrator roles in which they were trained and to which they had become accustomed. The nurses said their two most important roles are (1) integrator and (2) reviewer, and that after implementation of the new system, there was a significant decrease in their functioning in these roles. Physicians began to make mistakes that nurses had previously caught and corrected, such as ordering incorrect drugs or inaccurate dosages. In their new role, nurses tended to show less initiative in making treatment suggestions. What was lost was the second review and analysis by a trained professional—the second person had lost the overview perspective. On the other hand, some positive things did occur. Relieved of the orders paperwork, the nurses had two to three more hours per day to spend on hands-on patient care. Similar scenarios are likely to be repeated in behavioral health care.

Using this Scenario

This chapter presents both theoretical concepts and practical techniques for dealing with informatics change processes. Each of the concepts relate to this scenario, especially in terms of the role of behavioral health and its informatics in the modern healthcare organization.

Types of Change

Changes within an organization can often be identified as one of four types, which may overlap:

- *Operational*—changes in the way that business is conducted, such as the automation of a particular area
- *Strategic*—changes in the business direction, e.g., moving from an inpatient to a continuum of care focus
- *Cultural*—changes in the basic organizational philosophies by which the business is conducted, e.g., implementing a continuous quality improvement (CQI) system
- *Political*—changes in staffing occurring for various reasons such as top patronage job levels in government agencies.

These four types of change typically have impact at different levels of the organization. For example, operational changes tend to have their greatest repercussion at the lower levels of the organization, at the front line. Those at the upper levels may never notice changes that cause significant stress and turmoil to those attempting to implement the changes. Conversely, the impact of political change is typically felt at the higher organizational levels, where changes are typically not made for result-oriented reasons but for reasons such as partisan politics or internal power struggles. When these changes occur in a bureaucratic organization, the employees at the bottom rarely notice the changes at the top. Patients are seen and the floors are cleaned just as before. The key point is that performance was not the basis of the change; therefore, the performers are not affected.

Resistance to Change

People are most comfortable with the status quo unless it is inflicting discomfort. Even then, people will often resist change; "devil you know is better than the devil you don't know." It is a shock for inexperienced managers the first time they see subordinates resist even a change that they requested.

Resistance Against What?

There can be countless reasons for resistance to change in a given situation, thus the term resistance to change is often used very broadly. One of the first aspects that must be analyzed is the difference between

• resistance to a particular *change* and
• resistance to the perceived *changer(s)*.

In the first case, the resistance is directed against the changes in the system. In the second case, the resistance occurs because of negative feelings toward specific units, specific managers, or the organization in general; any change would be resisted just because of who or what is behind it. Both types of resistance have to be dealt with, but it is critical that we correctly identify the resistance category.

When a new behavioral health informatics system is introduced, three questions are very important to ask:

• What is the general organizational climate—positive or negative, cooperative or adversarial, etc.?
• What has been the nature of the process used to implement previous informatics systems?
• What has been the technical quality of the informatics systems previously implemented?

Whether or not we are new to an organization, we inevitably inherit the organizational climate and history. This negative "baggage" can be a frustrating burden that adds significantly to the challenge of successfully implementing a new system. On the other hand, the ability to meet this type of challenge is a differentiating quality of skilled implementers.

Intensity of Resistance

Resistance can vary in many ways, and perceptions regarding resistance can vary widely from one observer to another. One might perceive an end user who asks many questions as being very interested and actively seeking knowledge. Another might see the same person as a troublemaker who should just "shut up and listen!"

We can safely assume that every significant health informatics implementation is going to encounter some resistance; however, the intensity of resistance can vary widely. In an organization with a history of managing changes reasonably well and of decent morale, a significant number of people may be neutral toward a particular proposed systems change. However, there will still be a negative component, and at the very least this negative component must be managed and prevented from growing. In every situation, the proportions of positive, negative, and neutral may vary widely.

The Cast of Characters

For any given change, people occupy a wide range of roles that strongly influence their perceptions of the change and ultimately their reaction to it. Some people may have more than one role, or the roles may be unique. Unless we clearly identify both the players and their roles in any change situation, we risk making decisions and taking action based on generalizations that are not true for some of the key players. The following categories provide one way of looking at the various roles involved in an overall change process:

The *initiator* or instigator perceives the problem situation or opportunity and conceptualizes the change to be made in response.

The *approver* or funder is the power figure who okays and financially supports the proposed change.

The *champion* or cheerleader is the visible, enthusiastic advocate for the change. The champion constantly tries to rally support for the change and maintain that support during difficult periods.

The *facilitator* attempts to assist in smoothing the organizational change process. The facilitator is sometimes involved from the beginning, and sometimes is called in only for assistance once the change process has gone awry.

The *developer* or builder is responsible for the technical aspects of the change, e.g., developing the new informatics system. These aspects can range from the broad technical conceptualization to the narrowest of technical details.

The *installer* is responsible for implementing the change, including the necessary training and support activities.

The *doer* is the "changee," the person who has to work in the changed environment.

The *obstructionist* is a guardian of the status quo and typically conducts guerrilla warfare against the change. If the obstructionist is also a doer, the reason may arise from a personal fear of the change. However, the desire to obstruct may also arise from forces such political infighting, e.g., who gets the credit, or institutional conflicts, e.g., union resistance to a labor-saving system.

The *customer* is the end-beneficiary or victim of the change in terms of altered levels of service, cost, etc.

The *observer* does not perceive being immediately affected by the change, but instead observes with interest. These observations often affect strongly how the observer will react if placed in the doer role in the future.

The *ignorer* perceives that this change has no personal implications and is indifferent to it. In the broadest sense, this category also includes all those who are unaware of the change.

An overview term often applied to all these roles is *stakeholders*. With the exception of the ignorers, all the categories have some stake or interest in the quality of the change and the change implementation process. The roles are subject to change, especially during a change process that extends over time. For example, an initial ignorer might hear rumblings of discontent within the system and change to an observer, at least until the feelings of angst subside.

For those implementing change, the following steps are critical:

1. identify what roles stakeholders are occupying in the process;
2. identify what roles others involved in the process are playing, being careful to recognize multiple roles;
3. identify which role is speaking whenever communicating with those playing multiple roles; and
4. monitor throughout the process, and whether any roles are changing.

Magnitudes of Change

Change, like beauty, is in the eye of the beholder. A proposed change that upsets one person may be a welcome alleviation of boredom to another. The types and magnitudes of reaction are often difficult for an outsider to predict. When working with change and change management, it often helps to have a simple way of classifying the types and sizes of change.

Microchanges and Megachanges

A practical model that we frequently use divides changes into *microchanges* (differences in degree) and *megachanges* (differences in kind). Using an information system as an example, modifications, enhancements, improvements, and upgrades would typically be microchanges, while a new system or a major revision of an existing one would be a megachange. This scheme works well in communicating within organizations if we remember that one person's microchange is another person's megachange. Later in this chapter we present a more rigorous analysis of the magnitude of change that can be used if necessary.

Classic Change Theories

The rate of change in most organizations is escalating, and healthcare organizations—after a slow start—are no exception. The phrase *change management* has become fairly common in the literature on management. What is change management? How does it help people feel less threatened? How did it evolve? Why are people fixated on it today? What is a "change agent" or a change management person?

Change management is the process by which an organization achieves its vision. While traditional planning processes delineate the steps on the journey, change management attempts to facilitate that journey. Therefore, creating change starts with creating a vision for change and then empowering individuals to act as change agents to attain that vision. The empowered change management agents need plans that are (1) a total systems approach, (2) realistic, and (3) future oriented. Change management encompasses the effective strategies and programs to enable the champions to achieve the new vision. Today's change management strategies and techniques derive from the theoretical work of several pioneers in the change area.

Early Group Theories

In 1974, Watzlawick et al[5] published their now classic book, *Change: Principles of Problem Formation and Problem Resolution*. Theories about change had long existed. However, Watzlawick et al found that most of the theories of change were philosophical and derived from the areas of mathematics and physics. They selected two theories from the field of mathematical logic—the theory of groups and the theory of logical types—upon which to base their beliefs about change. Their goal of reviewing the theories of change was to explain the accelerated phenomenon of change that they were witnessing. Let us briefly look at the two theories that Watzlawick et al. reviewed to develop their change theory.

The more sophisticated implications of the *theory of groups* can be appreciated only by mathematicians or physicists. Its basic postulates concern the relationships between parts and wholes. According to the theory, a group has several properties, including members that are alike in one common characteristic. These members can be numbers, objects, concepts, events, or whatever else one wants to draw together in such a group, as long as they have at least one common denominator. Another property of a group is the ability to combine the members of the group in a number of varying sequences and have the same combinations. The theory of groups gives a model for the types of change that transcend a given system.

The *theory of logical types* begins with the concept of collections of "things" that are united by a specific characteristic common to all of them. For example, mankind comprises all individuals but is not a specific individual. Any attempt to change one in terms of the other does not work and leads to nonsense and confusion. For example, the economic behavior of the population of a large city cannot be understood in terms of the behavior of one person multiplied by four million. A population of four million people is both quantitatively and qualitatively different from an individual. Similarly, while the individual members of a species are usually endowed with very specific survival mechanisms, the entire species may race headlong toward extinction—and the human species is probably no exception.

The theory of groups gave Watzlawick et al the framework for thinking about the kind of change that can occur within a system that itself stays invariant. The theory of logical types is not concerned with what goes on inside a class, but gave the authors a framework for considering the relationship between member and class and the peculiar metamorphosis that is in the nature of shifts from one logical level to the next higher. From this, they concluded that there are two different types of change: one that occurs within a given system that itself remains unchanged, and one whose occurrence changes the system itself. For example, a person having a nightmare can do many things in his dream—hide, fight, scream, jump off a cliff, etc. However, no change from any one of these behaviors to another would terminate the nightmare. Watzlawick et al concluded that this is a first-order change. The one way out of a dream involves a change from dreaming to waking. Waking is no longer a part of the dream, but a change to an altogether different state. This is their second-order change as mentioned earlier.

First-order change is a variation in the way processes and procedures have been done within a given system, leaving the system itself relatively unchanged. Some examples are creating new reports, creating new ways to collect the same data, and refining existing processes and procedures.

Second-order change occurs when the system itself is changed. This type of change usually occurs as the result of a strategic change or a major crisis such as a threat to system survival. Second-order change involves a redefinition or reconceptualization of the business of the organization and the way it is to be conducted. In the medical area, fully changing from a paper medical record to an electronic medical record would represent a second-order change, just as automated teller machines redefined the way that banking functions are conducted.

These two orders of change represent extremes. First order involves doing better what we now do, while second order radically changes the core ways we conduct business or even the basic business itself.

A middle level seems to be missing from these two extremes. Golembiewski et al[6] added another level of change. They defined *middle-order change* as lying somewhere between the extremes of first- and second-order change. Middle-order change "represents a compromise; the magnitude of change is greater than first-order change, yet it neither affects the critical success factors nor is strategic in nature." An example of a middle-order change might be the introduction of an electronic mail system into an organization. There is an organization-wide impact, but there is no reconceptualization of the basic business. E-mail is more of a tool for operational and communications efficiency.

Some personality types welcome changes that they perceive will make their jobs easier while other personality types use their day-to-day work rituals to build their comfort zones. In the late 1960s, one unit in a medical center started to code all of their continuing medical education courses with International Classification of Diseases (ICD-9) codes. Even though these codes were never used and took a great deal of time to complete, the organization did not want to change the process as time passed because "we have always done it this way." The old process lasted through two directors. When a new director tried to change the process, there was resistance.

The most important question to an individual involved in any change process, regardless of the level or degree of change or the person's organizational position, is, "How will this affect me?" The most traumatic changes are of the second-order change type, but one person might perceive changes in the first or middle order as more traumatic than another person might perceive a second-order change. One of the challenges for the change manager is successfully managing these perceptions. How the change manager implements the process of change can have a decided effect on the resistance factors.

When Watzlawick et al's[5] book was published, many people were unfamiliar with the applications of theories of change into contemporary society; thus, the book was a major contribution to alternative ways of looking at the changes that occur daily. While Watzlawick et al comprehensively presented the theories of change and offered their model of levels of change, they did not offer practical day-to-day strategies. We are interested in the effective strategies for managing change and have reviewed many social science theories to determine the psychology behind the change management concepts and strategies that are used widely today. We believe that today's successful change management strategies emanate from several theories in the areas of psychology and sociology. Small group theories and field theories provide the antecedents of today's successful change management practices.

Small Group Theories

The *primary group* is one of the classical concepts of sociology, and many sociological theories focus on small-group analysis and the interaction process analysis. These theories outline and delineate small-group behavior. Small-group theories help us to understand not only how to make things more successful, but also how to analyze when things go wrong. For example, a practical application of small-group research was presented by Bales,[7] who applied small group principles to running a meeting and made the following suggestions:

- If possible, restrict committees to seven members.
- Place all members so they can readily communicate with every other member.
- Avoid committees as small as two or three if a perceived power problem between members is likely to be critical.
- Select committee members who are likely to participate in varying amounts. A group with all highly active participants or all minimally active participants will be difficult to manage.

An example of small-group behavior at work is a job candidate being interviewed by a number of people. Information is then collected from the interviewers and is shared with a search committee. The search committee selects their top candidate, and that person is hired. If the person hired does not work out, a member of the search committee may very well say, "I knew that Mary would not work out, but I didn't say anything because everyone seemed to like her."

Many of the changes that new technology brings are discussed, reviewed, and debated by people in a small-group framework. If negative sentiments about a product or service are stated by a member of the group who is an opinion leader, the less vocal people will often not challenge the dominant opinion. For example, a medium-sized organization was selecting a local area network (LAN) system. While the senior leader wanted one system, some of the other people had not only suggestions but also documentation about the qualities of another system. During the meeting to decide which system to purchase, the senior leader stated his views first and quite strongly. A couple of the lower-level staff members started to confront the senior person; however, when there was no support from any of the other people present, they did not express their strong preferences for their system of choice. When the system finally arrived, the senior leader's initial enthusiasm had dwindled. He then confronted the technology people as to why they had not made him aware of the shortcomings of the system selected.

These examples illustrate a key change management requirement: to effectively manage change, it is imperative for change agents to understand how people behave in groups and especially in small groups.

Field Theory

Kurt Lewin and his students are credited with combining theories from psychology and sociology into the field theory in social psychology.[8] Lewin focused his attention on motivation and the motivational concepts that underlie an individual's behavior. Lewin believed that there is tension within a person whenever a psychological need or an intention exists, and the tension is released only when the need or intention is fulfilled. The tension may be positive or negative. These positive and negative tension concepts were translated into a more refined understanding of conflict situations and, in turn, what Lewin called "force fields."

Lewin indicated that there are three fundamental types of conflict:

1. The individual stands midway between two positive goals of approximately equal strength. A classic metaphor is the donkey starving between two stacks of hay because of the inability to choose. In information technology, if there are two good systems to purchase or options to pursue, then we must be willing to choose.
2. The individuals find themselves between two approximately equal negative goals. This certainly has been a conflict within many organizations wishing to purchase or build a health informatics system. A combination of the economics, the avail-

able technologies, and the organizational issues may well mean that the organization's informatics needs cannot be satisfied with any of the available products—whether purchased or developed in-house. Thus, the decision makers must make a choice of an information system that they know will not completely meet their needs. Their choice will probably be the lesser of two evils.
3. The individual is exposed to opposing positive and negative forces. This conflict is very common in healthcare organizations today, especially regarding health informatics. This conflict usually occurs between the systems users and the information technology people or the financial people.

People can easily be overwhelmed by change, especially within large organizations where they may perceive they have little or no voice in, or control over, the changes they perceive are descending upon them. The typical response is fight or flight, not cooperation. Managers often interpret such human resistance to change as stubbornness or not being "on the team." This reaction solves nothing in terms of reducing resistance to change or gaining acceptance of it. Many managers do not accept that they are regarded as imposing "life-threatening" changes and establishing "no-win" adversarial relationships between management and those below in the organization.

Small-group theory is highly applicable in behavioral health informatics because of the way that medical environments are organized. The care of the patient or the education of students entails many small groups. These groups converse and share information and feelings, and strong opinion leaders can sway others to their way of thinking relatively easily.

Lewin's field theory diagrams the types of conflict situations commonly found in health care. In this way, the typical approach-avoidance forces can be visualized.[4] For example, "If I accept this new system, what will it mean to my job and me? Will I have a job? How will it change my role? Will this new system lessen my role?" These anxieties are very clear and very real to the people within the system. Remember: one person's microchanges are often another person's megachanges. So, as the system designers think they are making a minor change to enhance the total system, an individual end-user may see the change as a megachange and resist it vehemently. When designing the total people strategy for any system, it is important to involve the people from the very beginning and to clearly understand how groups function within the organization.

All of these social science theories assist the change management leader in understanding some of the underlying behavior issues as they bring health informatics technology into today's complex health systems.

Practical Change Management Strategies

Change management is the process of assisting individuals and organizations in moving from an old way of doing things to a new way. Therefore, a change process should both begin and end with a visible acknowledgment or celebration of the impending or just completed change. According to James Belasco,[9]

Our culture is filled with empowering transitions. New Year's Eve parties symbolize the ending of one year and the hope to be found in the one just beginning. Funerals are times to remember the good points of the loved one and the hope for new beginnings elsewhere. Parties given to retiring or leaving employees are celebrations of the ending of the employee's past status and the hope for the new opportunities to be found in the new status.

Based on our research, there is no single change management strategy that is effective in every situation. It is essential for the change management leader to take the time to know the desired state (vision-goal) and the particular organization and then to develop the appropriate strategies and plans to help facilitate the desired state.

Over the years we have evolved a core model for the major process of change management. There are many options within this model, but we believe that it is helpful for change leaders to have an overview map in mind as they begin to implement new information technology systems. The five-stage model that has proven effective for reducing barriers to technology change begins with an assessment and information-gathering phase.[10]

Assessment

The assessment phase of this model is the foundation for determining the organizational and user knowledge and ownership of the health informatics system that is under consideration. Ideally, this phase of the model begins even before the planning for the technological implementation of the new system. The longer the delay, the harder it will be to successfully manage the change and gain ultimate user ownership.

There are two parts to the assessment phase. The first is to *inform* all potentially affected people, in writing, of the impending change. This written information need not be lengthy or elaborate, but it will alert everyone to the changes in process.

The second part entails *collecting information* from those involved in the change by the use of both surveys and interviews. The survey instrument should be sent to randomly selected members of the affected group. One person in ten might be appropriate if the affected group is large. Five to ten open-ended questions should assess the individuals' current perceptions of the potential changes, their issues of greatest concern about these changes, and their suggestions to reduce those concerns. Recording and analyzing the responders' demographics will allow more in-depth analysis of the concerns raised by these potentially affected people.

In the personal face-to-face interviews with randomly selected people at all levels throughout the affected portions of the organization, it is important to listen to the stories the people are telling and to assess their positive and negative feelings about the proposed health informatics system. These interviews should help in ascertaining what each person envisions the future will be, both with and without the new system; what each interviewee could contribute to making that vision a reality; and how the interviewee could contribute to the future success of the new system. These interviews provide critical insights for the actual implementation plan. Often those people interviewed become advocates—and sometimes even champions—of the new system, thus easing the change process considerably.

An alternative or supplement to the one-on-one interviews is focus-group sessions. These allow anywhere from five to seven people from across the organization to share their feelings and ideas about the current system and new system.

Feedback and Options

The information obtained above must now be analyzed, integrated, and packaged for presentation to both top management and to those directly responsible for the technical implementation. This is a key stage for understanding the strengths and weaknesses of the current plans, identifying the major organizational areas of both excitement and resistance (positive and negative forces), identifying the potential stumbling blocks, understanding the vision the staff holds for the future, and reviewing the options suggested by the staff for making the vision come true. If this stage occurs early enough in the process, data from the assessment stage can be given to the new system developers for review.

When designing a model, this phase is important in order to establish that the organization learns from the inputs of its staff and begins to act strategically in the decision and implementation processes.

Strategy Development

This phase of the model allows those responsible for the change to use the information collected to develop *effective change strategies* from an organizational perspective. These strategies must focus on a visible, effective process to "bring on board" the affected people within the organization. This could include newsletters, focus groups, discussions, one-on-one training, and confidential "hand-holding"; the latter can be especially important for professionals such as physicians who may not wish to admit ignorance and/or apprehension about the new system.

Implementation

This phase of our model refers to the implementation of the change management strategies determined to be needed for the organization, not to the implementation of the new system. The implementation of the change strategies developed above must begin before the implementation of the new system. These behaviorally focused efforts consist of a series of steps, including informing and working with the people involved in a systematic and timely manner. This systematic progression toward the behavioral change desired and the future goals is important to each individual's acceptance of the new system. This is an effective mechanism for tying together the new technology implementation action plan with the behavioral strategies.

Reassessment

Six months after the new system is installed, a behavioral-effects data-gathering process should be conducted. This stage resembles the initial assessment stage— written surveys and one-on-one and/or focus group interviews. Data gathered from this stage allow measurement of the acceptance of the new system, which provides the basis for fine-tuning. This process also serves as input to the evaluation of the implementation process. It assures all the participants that their inputs and concerns are still valued and sought, even though the particular implementation has already occurred.

Conclusion

It is not always easy to know exactly why a particular person or group resists change. However, experience shows that an intelligent application of the basic five-step change model, coupled with a sound technological implementation plan, leads to more rapid and more productive introductions of technology into organizations. The process can be expensive in terms of time and energy but much less expensive than a technical system that never gains real user acceptance.

Perhaps most important, overall success requires an emotional commitment to success on the part of all involved. The staff must believe the project is being done for the right reasons—namely, to further the delivery of higher quality, cost-effective health care. If a project is generally perceived to be aimed at just "saving a quick buck" or boosting someone's ego or status, that project is doomed to fail.

An MCI television commercial depicts a book editor—faced with adapting to major informatics changes—commenting, "Art is constant; tools change." In the same vein, the ideals of behavioral health are a constant; the tools change. The challenge facing behavioral health informatics is to successfully implement those new tools in organizations that often do not welcome them.

Questions

1. Using your own words, define change management.
2. What might be some ways to help people celebrate remembering the past and moving to the future?
3. In the "Cast of Characters," which roles are nurses at various levels in the organizational hierarchy most likely to play? Why? What roles are nurses least likely to play? Why?
4. Why is the "feedback and options" phase so important in the change management model presented?
5. For the change scenario presented in this chapter, create a detailed change management plan that you think would lead to better results than those that were described in the scenario.

References

1. Høeg P. *Smilla's Sense of Snow*, trans. Nunnally T. New York: Dell, 1993.
2. Conner DR. Bouncing back. *Sky* 1994;30–34.
3. *Draft Proceedings of the International Medical Informatics Association Working Conference on the Organizational Impact of Informatics.* Cincinnati, OH: Riley Associates, 1993.
4. Lorenzi NM, Riley RT. *Organizational Aspects of Health Informatics: Managing Technological Change.* New York: Springer-Verlag, 1994:228–229.
5. Watzlawick P, Weakland JH, Fisch R. *Change: Principles of Problem Formulation and Problem Resolution.* New York: W. W. Norton, 1974.
6. Golembiewski RT, Billingsley K, Yeager S. Measuring change and persistence in human affairs: types of change generated by OD designs. *J Appl Behav Sci* 1976;12: 133–157.
7. Bales RF. In conference. *Harvard Business Review* 1954;32:44–50.
8. Deutsch M, Krauss RM. *Theories in Social Psychology.* New York: Basic Books, 1965.
9. Belasco JA. *Teaching the Elephant to Dance: Empowering Change in Your Organization.* New York: Crown, 1990.
10. Lorenzi NM, Mantel MI, Riley RT. Preparing your organizations for technological change. *Healthcare Informatics* 1990;7(12):33–34.

14
Evaluating the Impact of Behavioral Healthcare Informatics

NANCY M. LORENZI, NAAKESH A. DEWAN, AND ROBERT T. RILEY

One of the most challenging tasks in evaluating a behavioral health system is developing methods to isolate the effects of information technology within a dynamic environment such as behavioral health care. Many books and articles address the evaluation principles and methods. This chapter presents an overview of evaluation and its role in behavioral healthcare informatics system implementation. Behavioral health care has traditionally spent less on information technology as a percent of revenues than the medical and surgical fields. In the new millennium, the spending for informatics will increase, and evaluation of the return on investment must be undertaken if behavioral health care is to maximize its potential.

Many staff members in behavioral healthcare organizations struggle with understanding the impact of information technology on their organizations. They begin pointing to the lack of tangible results even before implementation projects are complete. Some people begin to question the implementation, and they express their anxiety by saying, "This isn't going to work." Others are impatient, worried about change. Many times organizations act to optimize short-term performance measures for new technology, but the process changes may take months or even longer to realize significant results.

The high-stake decisions linked to information technology implementation pressure the implementers to demonstrate that the new information technology makes a difference in their practices. Many behavioral practitioners fear that new technology efforts must produce measurable results in a relatively short time. The message about the expected effectiveness of technology, including outcome expectations, needs to be conveyed to the entire staff.

Today, evaluation research is used in the area of outcomes research, which has been conducted by people in the healthcare field. It is only fairly recently that health care has begun to accept and actively use outcomes research, which can be applied to the evaluation of the practice of medicine, with the intent that more informed decisions can be made by both the physician and the patient.

Critical Evaluation Issues

Evaluation Goals

In evaluating behavioral health informatics implementations, there are three critical questions. What is the correct target for the organization? How close did we come to the target that was selected? How many resources did it take to hit what was defined as the target? Keeping these three questions separate is critical in evaluation. If they are confounded in the evaluation process, the interpretation of any outcome is of questionable value.

Stakeholders

The stakeholders who support the new system need to be included in the evaluation process. This process includes identifying appropriate measurable indicators, and developing reliable instruments that will yield insightful and valid information about what makes information technology effective in behavioral health care. Stakeholders need information on how using information technology changes patient care, what the organizational impact of the information technology system will be, and what outcomes can be expected at different stages of the technology's implementation. The evaluation findings must be documented to satisfy diverse stakeholders' needs. Interest in technology's effectiveness is at an all-time high. Patients, and their families, want to know if they are improving and what their future outcomes will be. Administrators want to know if throughput is increasing with technology and if outcomes are improving. Funders, policymakers, and taxpayers want to know if information technology is promising to continue investing sufficiently in behavioral health care. Documenting and reporting evaluation data to meet these diverse stakeholders' questions presents evaluators with many challenges.

The difference in the data needs of policymakers/administrators and of practitioners is particularly acute. While policymakers/administrators want to see data on the effects of technology, practitioners need information that is tied to systemic practices. Policymakers/administrators tend to value reports documenting student achievement, while practitioners need reports documenting implementation outcomes to make sound decisions about their patient care plans. Many kinds of data are important, but data for policymakers fail to satisfy practitioners, and vice versa. The best hope of closing this gap lies in helping all stakeholders to see (1) the importance of information technology as an effective component of the behavioral medicine system, (2) the ways in which technology can and cannot make a difference, and (3) how innovative practices of behavioral medicine with technology require multiple measures to verify its impact.

Behavioral Health Care Practitioner

The role of the behavioral healthcare practitioner is crucial in evaluating the effectiveness of information technology. They must see evaluation as a reflective process to help improve their practice. Technology has the potential to revolutionize what behavioral healthcare practitioners do by several means, including interaction with some patients through technology. Information has added new breadth and depth to patient care by increasing the quality management. This, in turn, has the potential to transform the role of behavioral healthcare practitioners. Today practitioners need to know how to manage interactive group dynamics as well as information technological systems.

Implementing an innovation in behavioral healthcare practice can result in practice preceding policy. Some existing policies need to be transformed to match the new needs of practices using technology. One evaluation goal is to understand the conditions of technology use and to use that understanding for improving patient outcomes.

What Does Evaluation Entail?

Basically, evaluation and evaluation research are concerned with determining how well something works or how well something has been accomplished. That "something" could be an information system, a department within a hospital, or a particular service. Evaluation represents the application of social science research methods to discover information of importance about the program, practice, or department. This information can then be translated into future action.

Evaluation is undertaken to respond to areas of concern, such as

• analysis of an existing situation and development of a projected ideal,
• justification of a current or proposed activity, and
• analysis of the quality of an activity or operation.

One classic definition of evaluation is "the process of ascertaining the decision areas of concern, selecting appropriate information, and collecting and analyzing information in order to report summary data useful to decision makers in selecting among alternatives."[1] This definition of evaluation is based on the following assumptions:

• Evaluation is an information-gathering process.
• The information collected is used mainly to make decisions about alternative courses of action. Therefore, the collection and analysis procedures must be appropriate to the needs of the decision makers.
• Evaluation information should be carefully presented to the decision makers in a useful form, with great care taken to avoid confusing or misleading them.
• Different kinds of decisions will often require different kinds of evaluation procedures.[1]

Since healthcare organizations are in the business of trying to improve the human condition through a variety of organizational efforts, they are always making changes in services, departments, information systems, and so forth. An evaluation of those efforts is important to prove the value of the program or service. An evaluation of a behavioral health informatics system is needed not only to prove its value, but also to determine if the system is doing what was intended originally.

Are the information technology systems implemented in behavioral health care achieving their goals? Although this seems like a logical question, not everyone either wants to take the time to determine the answer or is interested in the answer. People may say, "The current system is working, and the technology is not available to do what the clinicians want." "We cannot ask the clinicians because we do not have the money for a new system anyway." "Leave well enough alone." Thus, those responsible for information systems sometimes do not see the need to evaluate since they have either limited desire or limited ability to change things.

There comes a point for most information system leaders when it is important to ask these questions:

- "How are we doing in general?"
- "Are we accomplishing what we set out to do?"
- "Are we meeting our end users' needs?"
- "Are we keeping current technically?"

A crisis may precipitate an evaluation inquiry, e.g., shortage of funds, competing needs, and obvious failures. The senior leaders want to know if they are getting their money's worth. In the case of a new information technology system, there is often a concern with learning whether the new system represents a good approach or if any changes are needed.

When there is interest in determining how well the information system is working, the evaluation can proceed by several routes. The processes are often foreign to those schooled primarily in the "hard sciences" that are used in working with variables that are more precisely measurable in physical terms. One way is through an impressionistic inquiry: an individual, a team, or a committee asks questions. Proceeding much as a journalist does, the investigators talk to the program director, staff members, and recipients of service (students, clients, and patients). They sit in on treatment sessions, attend meetings, look at reports, and usually in a few weeks or months come up with a report. Much useful information can be ferreted out in this way, but the procedure has obvious limitations. It relies heavily on what people are willing to reveal about the situation, including themselves. There is a noticeable difference if the investigators are from within versus outside the department. The journalistic inquiry depends, too, on the skill and insight of the investigators, and on their objectivity. If they are rushed, bland, or biased, their assessments can be wide of the mark. Perhaps the most significant drawback is to exclusively focus on what is happening at the present. Whatever the merit of its findings, the investigation usually tells little about outcomes, including what effect it has in helping participants achieve the goals that were originally undertaken.

Another assessment technique is to administer questionnaires or interviews that ask people's opinions about the program. Superficially, this appears more scientific and objective than the first type of investigation, and it does prevent the more patent intrusion of observers' biases. On the plus side, it also yields clues about program strengths and weaknesses. But again, as a method of evaluation, it is limited by what people divulge and by their immediate time perspective.[2]

The Link to Expectations

Information systems generally aim to provide people access to information that they need as accurately and rapidly as possible. Evaluation is the process needed to determine if the goals and expectations of the system were actually achieved. When beginning an informatics evaluation process, it is important (1) to have a baseline assessment of the current system, and (2) to link the evaluation to the comparison of outcomes to expectations. Before any organization decides to implement a new health information system, there are usually specific organizational expectations and goals for the new system. An evaluation will help organizations determine if the new behavioral health informatics system matches those initial systems expectations.

An evaluation process usually has three components: (1) an information gathering section, (2) an assessment of the information gathered, and (3) a decision or future action component. To better enable the organization to make future decisions, the evaluation process should be started at the very beginning of the development or acquisition process for a new health information system.

Baseline Analysis

To determine the real impact of any new system, it is important to measure where the organization is before the development or acquisition process begins. It is necessary to measure the state of the systems and the information flows before any action is taken. While the need for baseline information is important, practical reasons may prevent the baseline data from being collected. For example, the top managers may feel that immediate action is needed and that they cannot wait for a systematic evaluation. Another reason might be that the organization does not have the resources—money or people—to complete an evaluation of the current system.

One of the major benefits of a baseline evaluation is that it can help the organizational change leader and the senior leaders to thoroughly understand the current system. They can then determine if the change direction they are considering will meet the needs of the organization and its people. Another benefit is that the baseline information may be helpful after implementation to prevent spurious comparisons of the new system to the old one. This can come in handy if people start reminiscing about the "good old days" and how wonderful things were before this terrible new system was installed.

When evaluation is not considered until the installation of the new system is completed, the opportunity for an accurate baseline evaluation is lost. Those charged with postsystem evaluation must rely on retrospective reports, with all the risks of memory distortions, or on whatever documentary evidence happened to exist for other reasons at the time the decision to implement the new system was made. Such evidence is usually inadequate. Sometimes baseline measurements are incomplete simply because of lack of experience and foresight about what data might be needed later.

System Expectations

Before an organization makes a commitment to changing an information system or to installing a system where one does not exist, there are usually many hours of discussion and a clarification about the goals and expectations for the system. Organizational vision and needs are discussed, probable system costs are examined, and many organizational levels and people are consulted before final approval occurs.

To complete an effective evaluation of the new information system and the implementation process, it is essential that these realistic system expectations be clarified and used in the evaluation process as a measure of success or failure. The system expectations should be known to all involved in the system design and selection process. The expectations need to be written in simple declarative "capable of" statements, which are in turn used to develop evaluation questions and the evaluation methodology.

Evaluating the Implementation

The system implementation process is very important. Was the process smooth and without stress? Did the physicians and nurses actively participate and feel involved in the process? Did events happen as planned? What were the strengths and weaknesses of the manner in which the implementation occurred? These process-type issues are included in evaluating the actual implementation of a new behavioral health informatics system.

An actual first-hand account of what is being done is needed to evaluate the actions and events that occurred in the implementation process, especially if the system being implemented is for the total, complex health organization. Very often, the strategies listed initially differ from what happens in the "heat of battle." The person charged with the evaluation cannot assume that the plans and the actual implementation were as stated. There are a number of reasons for the possible discrepancy, including unclear perceptions or wishful thinking on the part of the staff and unrecognized conflict between people or groups. Evaluation is another reason why a dynamic planning and control process is so important. In addition to the direct planning benefits, such a process also provides a historic project trail for evaluation purposes.

One of the most difficult tasks in completing an evaluation study is finding the best techniques for understanding a process and the effects it has on people and systems and for estimating the degree to which observed phenomena approach the objectives of the program. This process is made easier by clear definitions of the goals and objectives. A practical problem of measurement in many studies is that of obtaining usable information. The application of evaluation techniques to the topic of an implementation process is usually costly and time-consuming, but important in order to redirect future efforts.

It is important to keep a record of the shifts, over time, in people's views. The views of some members of the behavioral medicine team will shift over the time of the project.

Assessment and developing new abilities for appraising change are a top priority among advocates of change. Learning to assess the consequences of significant change initiatives is a complex new territory, often neglected by leaders of those initiatives. In fact, assessment represents an opportunity for those advocating and championing change, particularly for line leaders. If they assume greater responsibility for assessment and measurement of their progress, they can make it a key strategy for accelerating learning. The key shift is to bring measurement and assessment into the service of learners, rather than have it feared as a tool for outside evaluators.

Evaluating the Quality of the System

After years of work, the health informatics system is implemented. Does the system do what it was originally designed to do? Is the system providing the type of information needed? What are the strengths and weaknesses of the system itself? The types of information that must be gathered in the evaluation of the system focus on how well the system performs and meets expectations.

The same techniques and issues that apply to the evaluation of the implementation process apply to the evaluation of the behavioral health informatics system. The collection, analysis, and presentation of data and information about the effectiveness of the new information technology–based system are important to determine if modifications are needed in the system or in the redesign of the current process/information flow. Recently, Dewan, Lorenzi, and Riley have developed a new benchmarking system for evaluating the quality of behavioral informatics systems and implementation. This benchmarking and evaluation system can be found on the Web at *bstpractice.com*. It asks users to first define the organizational climate and then in a longitudinal fashion rate the quality of the informatics implementation and the transformation that technology has made on the organization itself.

Time Delays

Time delays occur in implementing megachanges. The ultimate success or failure of the effort is based only on early results. Developing new capabilities is a matter of discipline and of regular practice with particular tools and methods, over the course of years. Those responsible for the information technology implementation can promote a realistic time period for others to realize and appreciate the resulting benefits.

What Do We Do with the Information?

The underlying belief in evaluation efforts is that the study of the data, information, and communication collected furnishes the basis for constant feedback and readjustment of activities within the complex organization. In earlier days, the concept was often referred to as "learning loops" or "feedback loops," but today the emphasis is on building what are known as "learning organizations."

The evaluation of complex organizations requires the formulation of objectives and criteria of accomplishment on a much broader scale. It is generally agreed that successful evaluation studies cannot be performed retrospectively, but rather must be built into the programs at their inception for true learning to take place. A number of considerations are advanced for such a position:

• When present from the beginning, the evaluation is less threatening, both because it seems to be part of the total process and because people come to feel they have had a hand in planning the evaluation.
• When skilled evaluators are an integral part of the planning phase of the system implementation, they can often help to improve the quality of the objectives as their attention is focused on the measurability of achievements.
• Experienced evaluators may be able to contribute substantively to the planning process by drawing on both their experiences and their knowledge of established social science findings. They may be able to suggest methods of known effectiveness and point out known difficulties in both the current operations and the system under development.
• Evaluators who are present from the start can follow the entire system and implementation process through planning, pretesting, and full-scale operations, thereby gathering information and keeping records of actual happenings.

Some organizations have established process action evaluation teams that may be made up of nurses, ward clerks, and other unit staff. The role of this team is to observe the day-to-day operations of the implementation process and to maintain a diary on the use and behavior of the system after it has been fully implemented. There are many ways for organizations to gather data. However, the key is using the data that have been gathered to make positive, proactive changes in the way systems are implemented within the organization and in the way that systems are designed and selected in the future.

Once the information from the evaluation is gathered and analyzed, it must be interpreted and summarized. The results of the evaluation are sometimes best communicated in small doses, allowing changes to be introduced gradually rather than abruptly. This approach reduces the resistance to any changes. If the people who did the evaluation remain as closely connected to the effort as possible and help the change leader and senior leaders interpret and implement the findings, the results of the evaluation are more likely to be adopted than if a report is dropped in the lap of the change manager with no provision made for explaining findings or helping implement action steps.

Conclusion

To evaluate means to assess value. Before the assessment can take place, the desired value must be understood. Evaluation criteria may include the following: "(1) To monitor a steady state so as to determine when a correction is necessary. (2) To identify alternatives in a problem (non-steady) situation and provide relevant information. (3) To weigh alternative courses of decision-making in terms of relative gains and losses. (4) To determine corrective action and the error-risks involved in various approaches to change."[3]

To study the problem of changing human behavior through evaluation, it is necessary to use applied and practical components of evaluation methods that can examine the topic at hand. The number of such components is limited, and the huge variety of behavior-change techniques utilized is variations on a few central themes. The heart of evaluation is listening to people and using their input to change the system in a meaningful way.

References

1. Alkin MC. Evaluation theory and development. *Eval Comment* 1969;2:2–7.
2. Weiss CH. *Evaluating Action Programs: Readings in Social Action and Education.* Boston: Allyn and Bacon, 1972.
3. Suchman EA. Action for what? A critique of evaluative research. In: O'Toole, R, ed. *Organization Management and Tactics of Social Research.* Cambridge: Schenkman, 1970.

Bibliography

Anderson JG. Evaluating clinical information systems: a step towards reducing medical errors. *MD Comput* 2000;17(3):21–22.
Dewan NA, Lorenzi NM. Behavioral health information systems evaluating readiness and user acceptance. *MD Comput* 2000;17(4):50–52.
Weiner M, Gress T, Thiemann DR, et al. Contrasting views of physicians and nurses about an inpatient computer-based provider order-entry system. *JAMIA* 1999;6(3):234–244.
Wood FB, Cid VH, Siegel ER. Evaluating Internet end-to-end performance: overview of test methodology and results. *JAMIA* 1998;5(6):528–545.

Index

Health Informatics Series
(formerly Computers in Health Care)

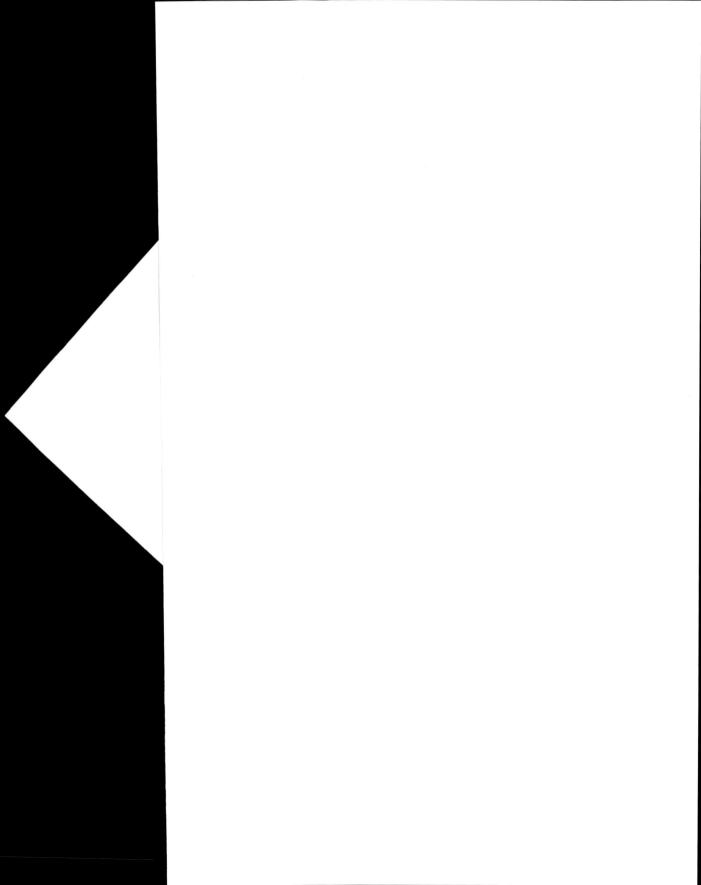

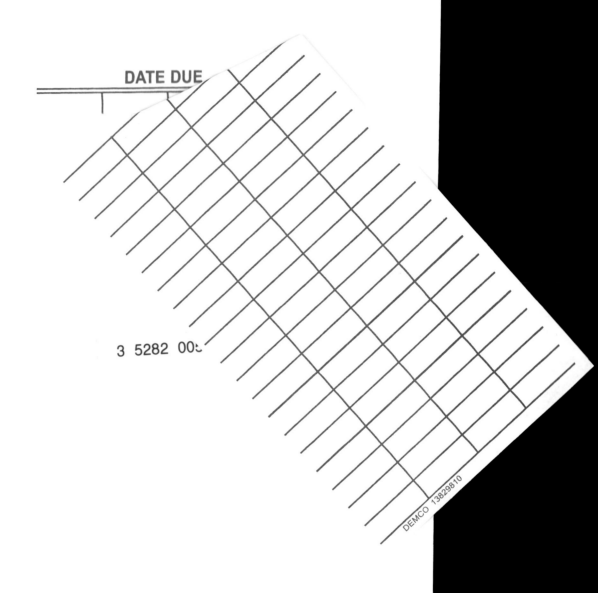

DATE DUE

3 5282 00